Reopening K–12 Schools During the

COVID-19 PANDEMIC

Prioritizing Health, Equity, and Communities

Enriqueta C. Bond, Kenne Dibner, and Heidi Schweingruber, *Editors*

Committee on Guidance for K–12 Education on Responding to COVID-19

Board on Science Education

Board on Children, Youth, and Families

Division of Behavioral and Social Sciences and Education

Standing Committee on Emerging Infectious Diseases and
21st Century Health Threats

A Consensus Study Report of

The National Academies of
SCIENCES · ENGINEERING · MEDICINE

THE NATIONAL ACADEMIES PRESS
Washington, DC
www.nap.edu

THE NATIONAL ACADEMIES PRESS   500 Fifth Street, NW   Washington, DC 20001

This activity was supported by contracts between the National Academy of Sciences and the Spencer Foundation (202100015) and the Brady Education Foundation (un-numbered). Any opinions, findings, conclusions, or recommendations expressed in this publication do not necessarily reflect the views of any organization or agency that provided support for the project.

International Standard Book Number-13: 978-0-309-68007-3
International Standard Book Number-10: 0-309-68007-7
Digital Object Identifier: https://doi.org/10.17226/25858
Library of Congress Control Number: 2020944328

Additional copies of this publication are available from the National Academies Press, 500 Fifth Street, NW, Keck 360, Washington, DC 20001; (800) 624-6242 or (202) 334-3313; http://www.nap.edu.

Suggested citation: *Reopening K–12 Schools During the COVID-19 Pandemic: Prioritizing Health, Equity, and Communities*. (2020). Washington, DC: The National Academies Press. https://doi.org/10.17226/25858.

The National Academies of
SCIENCES · ENGINEERING · MEDICINE

The **National Academy of Sciences** was established in 1863 by an Act of Congress, signed by President Lincoln, as a private, nongovernmental institution to advise the nation on issues related to science and technology. Members are elected by their peers for outstanding contributions to research. Dr. Marcia McNutt is president.

The **National Academy of Engineering** was established in 1964 under the charter of the National Academy of Sciences to bring the practices of engineering to advising the nation. Members are elected by their peers for extraordinary contributions to engineering. Dr. John L. Anderson is president.

The **National Academy of Medicine** (formerly the Institute of Medicine) was established in 1970 under the charter of the National Academy of Sciences to advise the nation on medical and health issues. Members are elected by their peers for distinguished contributions to medicine and health. Dr. Victor J. Dzau is president.

The three Academies work together as the **National Academies of Sciences, Engineering, and Medicine** to provide independent, objective analysis and advice to the nation and conduct other activities to solve complex problems and inform public policy decisions. The National Academies also encourage education and research, recognize outstanding contributions to knowledge, and increase public understanding in matters of science, engineering, and medicine.

Learn more about the **National Academies of Sciences, Engineering, and Medicine** at www.nationalacademies.org.

The National Academies of
SCIENCES · ENGINEERING · MEDICINE

Consensus Study Reports published by the National Academies of Sciences, Engineering, and Medicine document the evidence-based consensus on the study's statement of task by an authoring committee of experts. Reports typically include findings, conclusions, and recommendations based on information gathered by the committee and the committee's deliberations. Each report has been subjected to a rigorous and independent peer-review process and it represents the position of the National Academies on the statement of task.

Proceedings published by the National Academies of Sciences, Engineering, and Medicine chronicle the presentations and discussions at a workshop, symposium, or other event convened by the National Academies. The statements and opinions contained in proceedings are those of the participants and are not endorsed by other participants, the planning committee, or the National Academies.

For information about other products and activities of the National Academies, please visit www.nationalacademies.org/about/whatwedo.

v

Preface

When the Committee on Guidance for K–12 Education on Responding to COVID-19 began work on this study in May 2020, we were cognizant of the need to provide immediate, evidence-based guidance to education stakeholders around the nation on reopening schools for in-person learning. In order to offer guidance that would be useful in the planning process in advance of Fall 2020, we prepared a Consensus Study Report on a significantly abbreviated timeline. We could not have predicted the manner in which the discussions around the issue of reopening would explode while we completed this report.

As we discuss in this document, the research on the spread and mitigation of SARS-CoV-2 is expanding rapidly, leading to greater clarity on some topics while also pointing out new areas for investigation. Guidance documents for schools and districts are emerging at breakneck speed. In July 2020, opinion pieces are dominating the news media landscape, many of them staking out positions on either side of a "to reopen or not" debate and making bold claims about what is "safe." The politics of the moment are ablaze: one need only scan the headlines of U.S. newspapers to uncover the ways the politics around the question of reopening have overshadowed the scientific evidence.

The National Academy of Sciences (now expanded to the National Academies of Sciences, Engineering, and Medicine) was chartered by President Abraham Lincoln in 1863 to meet the government's urgent need for an independent adviser on scientific matters. Our organization is founded on the principle that independent guidance based on scientific evidence is essential for making sound policy. Development of that guidance needs to focus on interpreting scientific research without political influence: essentially, independence is necessary to ensure the integrity of the guidance. Furthermore, as the committee refers to in the Epilogue of this report, we know that evidence and data do not provide policy direction on their own: evidence and data must be interpreted, and these interpretations are never neutral. For this reason, the consensus study process at the National Academies demands that multiple perspectives are brought to bear on the available evidence: while "neutrality" is never possible, including multiple perspectives at the table can support an interpretation of the evidence that reflects the concerns of multiple constituencies and is as independent from individual bias as possible.

The Committee on Guidance for K–12 Education on Responding to COVID-19 has used this consensus study process to make sense of the best available evidence related to the transmission of SARS-CoV-2 while considering the contexts of schools and districts, and how best to maintain the health and well-being of children, school staff, and their broader communities. To the best of our ability, we have attempted to articulate guidance that will support decision-makers in doing the extremely challenging work of understanding and weighing risk, leveraging local assets, and balancing constraints in local resources. We have done this while new evidence is made available daily, and we recognize that the guidance contained in this report will need to be continually revisited as the science emerges around transmission and mitigation. Ultimately, we have written a report that puts science—what we know, as well as what we do not—at the center of the decision to reopen schools.

Given the urgent need for immediate guidance in advance of the impossibly challenging decisions ahead, the committee is acutely aware of the limitations in existing evidence. We know that one size does not fit all, and that every district will need to undertake a process that involves families, administrators, experts, and community leaders in the difficult task of how to redesign and reimagine what schools will look like in these uncertain times. We hope this report can offer support to education stakeholders around the nation as they make these deeply challenging decisions.

Enriqueta C. Bond, *Chair*
Kenne Dibner, *Study Director*
Committee on Guidance for K–12 Education
on Responding to COVID-19

Acknowledgments

This Consensus Study Report was reviewed in draft form by individuals chosen for their diverse perspectives and technical expertise. The purpose of this independent review is to provide candid and critical comments that will assist the National Academies of Sciences, Engineering, and Medicine in making each published report as sound as possible and to ensure that it meets the institutional standards for quality, objectivity, evidence, and responsiveness to the study charge. The review comments and draft manuscript remain confidential to protect the integrity of the deliberative process.

We thank the following individuals for their review of this report: Claire L. Barnett, Executive Director, Healthy Schools Network; Richard E. Besser, President and CEO, Robert Wood Johnson Foundation; Xavier Botana, Superintendent, Portland School District, Portland, ME; Catherine P. Bradshaw, Research and Faculty Development, Curry School of Education, University of Virginia; David V.B. Britt, Retired President and Chief Executive Officer, Sesame Workshop; Benjamin Cowling, School of Public Health, The University of Hong Kong; Kathryn M. Edwards, Department of Pediatrics, Vanderbilt University School of Medicine; Thomas V. Inglesby, Bloomberg School of Public Health and School of Medicine, Johns Hopkins University; Jennifer O'Day, Institute Fellow, American Institutes for Research; Diane S. Rentner, Center on Education Policy, Graduate School of Education and Human Development, The George Washington University; Jerry Roseman, Environmental Science and Occupational Safety and Health, Philadelphia Federation of Teachers; and Megan M. Tschudy, Department of Pediatrics, Johns Hopkins University School of Medicine.

Although the reviewers listed above provided many constructive comments and suggestions, they were not asked to endorse the conclusions or recommendations of this report nor did they see the final draft before its release. The review of this report was overseen by Adam Gamoran, President, W.T. Grant Foundation, and Maxine Hayes, School of Medicine and School of Public Health, University of Washington. They were responsible for making certain that an independent examination of this report was carried out in accordance with the standards of the National Academies and that all review comments were carefully considered. Responsibility for the final content rests entirely with the authoring committee and the National Academies.

The committee's work benefited greatly from multiple outside experts who volunteered generously to share their expertise with the committee (see Appendix A). We especially thank the study sponsors—the Spencer Foundation, the Brady Education Foundation, and the National Academies' Standing Committee on Emerging Infectious Diseases and 21st Century Health Threats—for their commitment to this work.

It was a great privilege to work with such dedicated committee members who thoroughly engaged in the study and contributed significant time and effort to this very compressed endeavor. This committee was fortunate to work with a diligent and outstanding team of National Academies of Sciences, Engineering, and Medicine staff: thank you to Kenne Dibner, for her expert direction of this study from beginning to end. We thank Board on Science Education Director Heidi Schweingruber for her visionary leadership in conceiving of this study as well as her steadfast commitment to both substance and detail in all aspects of completing this report. We thank Leticia Garcilazo Green for her excellent work in both research and report production. We thank Matthew Lammers for his invaluable administrative work for this project, and Mary Filardo for her ongoing and insightful contributions as a consultant to the committee. Kirsten Sampson Snyder of the DBASSE staff deftly guided us through the National Academies review process, and Rona Briere and Allie Boman provided invaluable editorial assistance.

Enriqueta C. Bond, *Chair*

Contents

Summary

The COVID-19 pandemic has presented unprecedented challenges to the nation's K–12 education system. The rush to slow the spread of the virus led to closures of schools across the country, with little time to ensure continuity of instruction or to create a framework for deciding when and how to reopen schools. States, districts, and schools are now grappling with the complex and high-stakes questions of whether to reopen school buildings and how to operate them safely if they do reopen. These decisions need to be informed by the most up-to-date evidence about the SARS-CoV-2 virus that causes COVID-19; about the impacts of school closures on students and families; and about the complexities of operating school buildings as the pandemic persists.

In response to this need for evidence-based guidance, the Board on Science Education of the National Academies of Sciences, Engineering, and Medicine, in collaboration with the National Academies' Board on Children, Youth, and Families and Standing Committee on Emerging Infectious Disease, convened the Committee on Guidance for K–12 Education on Responding to COVID-19. The committee was tasked with providing guidance on the reopening and operation of elementary and secondary schools for the 2020–2021 school year. This report documents the committee's findings, conclusions, and recommendations with respect to (1) what is known (and not known) about COVID-19, (2) what is necessary to know about schools in order to make decisions related to COVID-19, (3) how determinations about reopening schools and staying open can best be made, and (4) strategies for mitigating the spread of COVID-19 in schools.

EQUITY AND REOPENING SCHOOLS

The committee was particularly concerned about how the persistent inequities of the education system might interact with similar disparities in health outcomes and access in ways that could devastate some communities more than others. Every choice facing states, districts, and schools is being made against the backdrop of entrenched economic and social inequities made more visible by the disparate impacts of the pandemic on Black, LatinX, and Indigenous communities. Without careful attention, plans to reopen schools could exacerbate these inequities.

COVID-19, CHILDREN, AND TRANSMISSION

Evidence to date suggests that children and youth (aged 18 and younger) are at low risk of serious, long-term consequences or death as a result of contracting COVID-19. However, there is insufficient evidence with which to determine how easily children and youth contract the virus and how contagious they are once they do. Similarly, while some measures—such as physical distancing, avoiding large gatherings, handwashing, and wearing masks—are clearly important for limiting transmission, there is no definitive evidence about what suite of strategies is most effective for limiting transmission within a school setting when students, teachers, and other staff are present. The fact that evidence is inadequate in both of these areas—transmission *and* mitigation—makes it extremely difficult for decision-makers to gauge the health risks of physically opening schools and to create plans for operating them in ways that reduce transmission of the virus.

WEIGHING THE RISKS OF BUILDING CLOSURES

Keeping schools closed to in-person learning in Fall 2020 poses potential educational risks. Students of all ages benefit from in-person learning experiences in ways that cannot be fully replicated through distance learning. The educational risks of extended distance learning may be higher for young children and children with disabilities. In addition, without careful implementation, virtual learning alone runs the risk of exacerbating disparities in access to high-quality education across different demographic groups and communities.

Opening school buildings to some extent in Fall 2020 may provide benefits for families beyond educating children and youth. Working caregivers would have affordable, reliable child care for school-age children, and families would be better able to access services offered through the school, such as provision of meals and other family supports (e.g., mental health services, school-based health services).

If and when schools reopen, staffing is likely to be a major challenge. A significant portion of school staff are in high-risk age groups or are hesitant to return to in-person schooling because of the health risks. In addition, some of the strategies for limiting the transmission of COVID-19 within schools, such as maintaining smaller class sizes and delivering both in-person and virtual learning, will require additional instructional staff.

THE DECISION TO REOPEN

While many guidance documents for reopening schools exist, many state-level guidance documents do not explicitly call on districts to reopen schools; rather they pose a series of questions for districts to consider in making decisions about reopening. This approach to providing guidance allows for regional variation and flexibility. However, it also leaves district leaders with a tremendous responsibility for making judgments about the risks of reopening while also responding to the needs of students, families, and staff.

Weighing all of the relevant factors to arrive at a decision about reopening and staying open involves simultaneously considering the public health risks, the educational risks, and other potential risks to the community. This kind of risk assessment requires expertise in public health, infectious disease, and education as well as clear articulation of the community's values and priorities. It also requires a protocol for monitoring data on the virus to track community spread. To ensure that the process of reopening schools is reflective of the community's needs and values and attends effectively to the multiple (and often conflicting) priorities of the numerous stakeholders, schools and districts will need to take care to engage a range of perspectives in the decision-making process.

IMPLEMENTING MITIGATION STRATEGIES

Reopening school buildings will be contingent on implementing a set of mitigation strategies that limits transmission of the virus. The existing guidance documents offer an extensive list of potential strategies but little guidance on how districts and schools can or should prioritize them. Many of the mitigation strategies currently under consideration (such as limiting classes to small cohorts of students or implementing physical distancing between students and staff) require substantial reconfiguring of space, purchase of additional equipment, adjustments to staffing patterns, and upgrades to school buildings. The financial costs of consistently implementing a number of potential mitigation strategies is considerable. While some highly resourced districts with well-maintained buildings may be able to implement most of the strategies, many schools and districts will need additional financial support to institute and maintain mitigation measures. Costs are a particular concern due to the budget cuts resulting from the economic impact of the pandemic.

Poor-quality school buildings (i.e., those that have bad indoor air quality, are not clean, or have inadequate bathroom facilities) complicate reopening and may make it difficult for school districts to implement the recommended health and safety measures. This poses a problem for equitable implementation of the strategies as children and youth from low-income families disproportionately attend schools with poor-quality facilities.

Finally, even if all of the mitigation strategies are in place and well implemented, it is impossible to completely eliminate the risk of COVID-19 in schools. Therefore, it is incumbent on school officials, in association with local public health authorities, to plan for the possibility that one or more students, teachers, or staff will contract COVID-19.

RECOMMENDATIONS

The committee formulated a set of recommendations designed to help districts and schools successfully navigate the complex decisions around reopening school buildings, keeping them open, and operating them safely. In its final recommendation, the committee identifies four areas of research that are urgently needed to fill the existing gaps in evidence: (1) the role of children in transmission of SARS-CoV-2, (2) the role of reopening schools in the spread of SARS-CoV-2 in communities, (3) the role of airborne transmission of COVID-19, and (4) the relative effectiveness of different mitigation strategies in schools.

Recommendation 1: *The Decision to Reopen*
Districts should weigh the relative health risks of reopening against the educational risks of providing no in-person instruction in Fall 2020. Given the importance of in-person interaction for learning and development, districts should prioritize reopening with an emphasis on providing full-time, in-person instruction in grades K–5 and for students with special needs who would be best served by in-person instruction.

Recommendation 2: *Precautions for Reopening*
To reopen during the pandemic, schools and districts should provide surgical masks for all teachers and staff, as well as supplies for effective hand hygiene for all people who enter school buildings.

Recommendation 3: *Partnerships Between School Districts and Public Health Officials*
Local public health officials should partner with districts to
- assess school facilities to ensure that they meet the minimum health and safety standards necessary to support COVID-19 mitigation strategies;
- consult on proposed plans for mitigating the spread of COVID-19;
- develop a protocol for monitoring data on the virus in order to (a) track community spread and (b) make decisions about changes to the mitigation strategies in place in schools and when future full school closures might be necessary;
- participate in shared decision-making about when it is necessary to initiate closure of schools for in-person learning; and
- design and deliver COVID-19–related prevention and health promotion training to staff, community, and students.

Recommendation 4: *Access to Public Health Expertise*
States should ensure that in portions of the state where public health offices are short-staffed or lack personnel with expertise in infectious disease, districts have access to the ongoing support from public health officials that is needed to monitor and maintain the health of students and staff.

Recommendation 5: *Decision-Making Coalitions*
State and local decision-makers and education leaders should develop a mechanism, such as a local task force, that allows for input from representatives of school staff, families, local health officials, and other community interests to inform decisions related to reopening schools. Such a cross-sector task force should
- determine educational priorities and community values related to opening schools;
- be explicit about financial, staffing, and facilities-related constraints;
- determine a plan for informing ongoing decisions about schools;
- establish a plan for communication; and
- liaise with communities to advocate for needed resources.

Recommendation 6: *Equity in Reopening*
In developing plans for reopening schools and implementing mitigation strategies, districts should take into account existing disparities within and across schools. Across schools, plans need to address disparities in school facilities, staffing shortages, overcrowding, and remote learning infrastructures. Within schools, plans should address disparities in resources for students and families. These issues might include access to technol-

ogy, health care services, ability to provide masks for students, and other considerations.

Recommendation 7: *Addressing Financial Burdens for Schools and Districts*
Schools will not be able to take on the entire financial burden of implementing the mitigation strategies. Federal and state governments should provide significant resources to districts and schools to enable them to implement the suite of measures required to maintain individual and community health and allow schools to remain open. Under-resourced districts with aging facilities in poor condition will need additional financial support to bring facilities to basic health and safety standards. In addition, State Departments of Education should not penalize schools by withholding statewide school funding formula monies for student absences during the COVID-19 pandemic.

Recommendation 8: *High-Priority Mitigation Strategies*
Based on what is currently known about the spread of COVID-19, districts should prioritize mask wearing, providing healthy hand hygiene solutions, physical distancing, and limiting large gatherings. Cleaning, ventilation, and air filtration are also important, but attending to those strategies alone will not sufficiently lower the risk of transmission. Creating small cohorts of students is another promising strategy.

Recommendation 9: *Urgent Research*
The research community should immediately conduct research that will provide the evidence needed to make informed decisions about school reopening and safe operation. The most urgent areas for inquiry are
- children and transmission of COVID-19,
- the role of reopening schools in contributing to the spread of COVID-19 in communities,
- the role of airborne transmission of COVID-19, and
- the effectiveness of different mitigation strategies.

1

K–12 Schools and COVID-19: Context and Framing

The COVID-19 pandemic has presented unprecedented challenges to the nation's K–12 education system. The rush to respond to the pandemic led to closures of school buildings across the country, with little time to ensure continuity of instruction or to create a framework for deciding when and how to reopen schools. States, districts, and schools are now grappling with responding to the rapidly changing situation while also trying to address the consequences of disruptions to schooling and ensure the health and safety of students, families, and staff. The crisis is ongoing: even as schools are slated to begin a new academic year in Fall 2020, the United States will still be in the midst of the COVID-19 pandemic with no available vaccine. School systems need guidance as the pandemic continues to unfold, and communities need evidence-based information to support appropriate decisions in the midst of often conflicting medical, social, and political pressures. Although intended to be helpful, contradictory messages—from education leaders, from nongovernmental organizations, from health officials, from politicians, from parents and families—complicate decision-making for everyone.

In addition, the impact of the pandemic has laid bare the deep, enduring inequities that afflict the nation in a wide range of areas, including the education system. The persistent disparities within the education system have come into sharp focus as schools and districts have grappled with how to provide meaningful learning experiences for all students as well as how to continue providing essential supports to families and communities, including meals and access to health care services while they operate their schools remotely. Plans for physically reopening and operating schools

7

during the pandemic must address how to provide equitable access to instruction and services for all children and families.

STUDY SCOPE AND APPROACH

In response to the need for evidence-based guidance to support education decision-makers, the Board on Science Education of the National Academies of Sciences, Engineering, and Medicine, in collaboration with the Academies' Board on Children, Youth, and Families and the Standing Committee on Emerging Infectious Disease, convened an expert committee to provide guidance on the reopening and safe operation of elementary and secondary schools for the 2020–2021 school year (see Box 1-1).

The Committee on Guidance for K–12 Education on Responding to COVID-19 included members with a range of expertise that included education administration and policy, educational equity, school facilities, pediatrics, public health, and epidemiology. The committee met virtually five times over a 4-week period. To augment its own expertise, the committee heard testimony from outside experts on equity in education, child development, state education policy, school facilities, post-COVID inflammatory syndrome, and SARS-CoV-2 transmission in children. For more information about the committee's process for gathering and assessing evidence, see Appendix A.

One of the primary tasks facing National Academies committees is to determine the bounds of its statement of task. Accordingly, the committee made judgments about the scope of its work.

First, although the subject of this report is reopening K–12 schools,[1] this committee was not tasked with providing guidance on how to support student learning during the pandemic. To the extent that distance learning experiences are considered an alternative to in-person schooling or one component of a potential plan for reopening schools, the committee did consider the evidence on the outcomes of distance learning experiences. However, the committee was not tasked with drawing conclusions or making recommendations about how schools can support learning or address disruptions to student learning during this time.

Second, the committee determined that, given the short timeline for producing this report, an exhaustive, systematic review of all available guidance documents for schools and districts was not feasible. Since April 2020 and throughout the time the committee was developing the guidance

---

[1]In the majority of schools in the United States, schools did not "close" so much as transition to distance learning strategies. In this report, the committee notes that it uses the term "reopening schools" as shorthand to refer to reopening of school buildings for in-person learning in Fall 2020.

BOX 1-1
Statement of Task

The National Academies of Sciences, Engineering, and Medicine proposes an ad hoc committee to provide states and districts with guidance about whether and how to safely reopen schools in the 2020–2021 school year. The committee will write a report drawing on evidence from epidemiology, public health, education, and the social and behavioral sciences. The report will provide guidance on the health-related issues for safely reopening schools and the practices that should be implemented in order to maintain and monitor the health of staff and students. The report will address questions that have emerged from the planning efforts of state and district officials which are currently under way. The committee will address the following questions:

1. What indicators can state and district leaders use to determine if it is safe to reopen schools?
2. When schools reopen, what are the practices for maintaining and monitoring the health of staff and students that will be effective and practical? What are the risks and trade-offs if some practices cannot be adopted, or can only be partially adopted?
3. How can safety decisions and practices avoid reinforcing existing inequities in education instruction and facilities? Can new safety practices help reduce inequities?
4. How should affordability be assessed in relation to mitigation recommendations?
5. What provisions should be put in place for high-risk staff and students?
6. How will school mitigation be equitably adhered to?
7. How should the health and safety practices take into account the needs of students with disabilities?

in this report, numerous documents offering recommendations for school reopening have been released. These include guidance from the Centers for Disease Control and Prevention (CDC), from national education organizations such as the Council of Chief State School Officers, from researchers in academia (for example, The Johns Hopkins University's Center for Health Security), from individual states, and from professional organizations and teachers' unions. These guidance documents vary in the extent to which they focus on best practices for public health, the practical concerns of implementation in reopening and operating schools, the needs of students, and the needs of the education workforce. The nature of the evidence base grounding these documents also varies: as of this writing, many critical pieces of the COVID-19 puzzle remained missing. There still was limited evidence and no consensus on the extent to which children—particularly those who are infected but without symptoms—can transmit the virus to others, or on how effective the various strategies schools might employ to mitigate the transmission of SARS-CoV-2 might be. The committee examined the available guidance documents and looked for commonalities. As discussed in depth in this report, the committee was repeatedly struck by the lack of definitive direction for stakeholders in these documents, which effectively leaves school districts on their own to make judgments about reopening and operating schools.

Indeed, the committee found that proliferation of guidance documents was creating confusion at all levels about how to make sense of the varying perspectives on whether and how to reopen schools for in-person learning. The guidance in this report is intended to provide a framework for use by education leaders as they make high-stakes political and practical decisions about reopening schools for the 2020–2021 school year: to the extent possible, we attempted to formulate recommendations that would assist stakeholders in determining not only *whether* to reopen schools but also *how* to reopen schools. The committee recognizes the challenges faced by many schools with respect to operationalizing a number of the reopening strategies considered in this report, and where possible has attempted to comment directly on the relationship between feasibility and effectiveness. Ultimately, the goal is to integrate the most up-to-date evidence from medicine and public health with evidence about what is best for children and youth in view of the political and practical realities in schools and communities.

Because of the need to help stakeholders make sense of *whether* and *how* to reopen schools described above, the committee decided to structure this report in a way that would give readers both background about the challenges on the table as well as a series of tools for addressing those challenges. This decision lent itself to a report organization (described at the end of this chapter) that does not respond item-by-item to the questions posed in the statement of task. Rather than recapitulate the questions delineated above, the committee has integrated its responses to the statement of task into a broader narrative that describes the current context of the COVID-19 pandemic, how the pandemic has affected education in the United States, and our consideration of how decision-makers should proceed. In order to assist readers, we have included a sentence at the outset of each chapter that points to the parts of the statement of task addressed in the respective chapter. Where limited evidence has hindered our ability to respond to the posed questions, we have tried to identify additional research needs.

Finally, this report is not intended to supplant existing guidance documents from government agencies such as the CDC and state departments of education. In responding to the statement of task, the committee has written a report that applies multiple scholarly perspectives to the most current evidence on the transmission of SARS-CoV-2 so that education stakeholders can make informed decisions about reopening schools. Where possible, this report offers commentary intended to shed light on the challenges embedded in these decision-making processes, but stakeholders will need to review all relevant guidance documents in concert with one another in formulating cogent plans.

EQUITY AND COVID-19

As the committee interpreted the statement of task, it became clear that issues of equity are among the chief challenges facing stakeholders as they decide whether and how to reopen schools. The ability of public schools to meet the needs of their communities is contingent upon the resources available to them: as we discuss throughout this report, many schools and districts are ill equipped to provide even the most basic services to students and families. More urgently, the onset of the COVID-19 pandemic has served to exacerbate these existing inequities by cutting children and families off from the resources that do exist. While many schools and districts have been able to leverage community resources to ensure that students are fed and cared for during the pandemic, there is no question that the shuttering of school buildings—and the consequent reliance on remote learning strategies—has meant that students are experiencing even more profound educational inequity than was the case prior to COVID-19.

At the same time, the COVID-19 pandemic has exacerbated ongoing challenges facing the U.S. health care system. There are significant, long-standing disparities in both individual and community health outcomes by education, income, race/ethnicity, geography, gender, neighborhood, disability status, and citizenship status (National Academies of Sciences, Engineering, and Medicine [NASEM], 2017). These disparities arise from social, economic, environmental, and structural disparities that contribute to intergroup differences in health outcomes across different communities. The root causes of health inequities include the forces and structures that organize the distribution of power and resources differentially depending on race, gender, class, and other dimensions of individual and group identity (NASEM, 2017). As discussed later in this report, the COVID-19 pandemic has only deepened these disparities.

In this political and public health context, the long-standing inequities in education and health outlined above have the potential to compound each other in ways that could be catastrophic for some communities. As described later in this report, the communities most devastated by COVID-19 are often also the same communities with inadequately resourced schools. Thus, it is clear that for some communities, it will be incumbent upon stakeholders considering the risks, trade-offs, and costs of reopening schools to address these equity issues head on in determining effective strategies for responding to COVID-19.

Finally, the committee has written this report in the same moment as the Black Lives Matter protests. Driven by outrage around the murders of Black individuals by police, people have taken to the streets to protest the systemic racism woven into the fabric of U.S. society. Although this committee was not tasked with commenting on racial justice, it is not possible to talk about the role of schools in society without also acknowledging the long history of schools in perpetuating and reproducing systemic racism. This backdrop cannot be ignored as a contributing factor in how the nation will make sense of the many issues surrounding the reopening of schools.

THE QUESTION OF REOPENING

Decisions around how to reopen schools are among the most complex and consequential of the pandemic. When the outbreak in the United States intensified in March, schools were among the first community activities to close physically, in recognition of their role as community gathering places and the priority of protecting children.

More is now known about COVID-19 than was the case when the decision to close schools physically and move to distance learning was made, but there is still more to learn. Thus far, the science has suggested that children are at lower risk of severe illness relative to adults, and many infections in children are either asymptomatic or very mild. However, the extent to which children with asymptomatic or subclinical infection are able to transmit the virus to others remains unknown. If children do transmit the disease efficiently, as they do with influenza, for example, physically reopening schools could accelerate the transmission of COVID-19 in a community.

Data needed to answer this and other important questions are unlikely to be available by the time the decision to reopen will have to be made. Regardless of these decisions, however, the committee emphasizes that so long as the COVID-19 pandemic persists, there cannot be 100 percent safety in reopening schools for in-person learning. Given this, school systems and their surrounding communities will have to weigh the risks and uncertainties of reopening for in-person learning against the educational and social risks and challenges associated with continuing to educate and support students using a distanced model.

REPORT PURPOSE AND AUDIENCES

This report is intended primarily to provide guidance for those tasked with setting rules and parameters around school reopening and determining strategies for mitigating the transmission of COVID-19. The report is intended to provide insight for decision-makers especially concerned with weighing issues of health and safety alongside educational priorities and organizational conditions. Because of the nature of how schools are governed in the United States, the committee recognizes that the entity ultimately responsible for the final decisions around whether and how to reopen schools will vary across the country. For this reason, the committee wrote this report with multiple stakeholders in mind, and we expect this report will be useful to school administrators, teachers, and other relevant school staff who are seeking such guidance. The report should also be useful for policy makers and leaders at both the state and district levels, including governors, state superintendents, tribal leaders, and school board members. Other intended audiences include parents and community members who are directly affected by these decisions.

While the committee recognizes that many state, district, and school-based decisions related to school reopening are likely to be under way (if not completed) by the time of this report's publication, we also recognize the dynamic reality of decisions around COVID-19. That is, given the constantly shifting nature of the regional spread of the virus, ongoing demand for state and local resources, and the myriad competing demands and priorities of school stakeholders, the process of assessing both whether and how to reopen schools is likely to be ongoing. Thus, the committee prepared this report with an eye toward developing a framework that would enable decision makers to continually revisit their decisions as circumstances change and new needs and constraints arise.

Moreover, the committee recognizes that the answers to these questions are, to a large extent, contingent upon who is included in the process of answering them. Later in this report, we address critical considerations concerning which stakeholders should be engaged in making decisions for states, districts, and schools, and attempt to identify where in the education system decisions can and should be made.

REPORT ORGANIZATION

Chapter 2 provides an overview of the most up-to-date evidence about the spread of COVID-19, the course of the virus in children and youth (aged 4–18), and current understanding of the effectiveness of various public health measures for protecting individual and community health.

Chapter 3 examines the important role of schools in communities and the development of children and youth at different ages. Particular attention is given to the critical importance of considering the varying needs of different communities and the deep, structural inequities in the U.S. education system in making decisions about school reopening.

Chapter 4 integrates the evidence from Chapters 2 and 3 to provide guidance on how to determine whether schools should reopen for in-person operation in Fall 2020 and conversely whether additional closures may be needed. The discussion in this chapter responds to questions 1 and 3 in the committee's statement of task (Box 1-1).

Chapter 5 focuses on the range of strategies schools can and should use to maintain individual and community health once they reopen (whether partially or fully) for in-person learning. Strategies are considered from the perspective of what is most effective for maintaining health, what is practical and affordable for schools to adopt, and how a strategy can be implemented equitably. This chapter responds to questions 2, 3, 4, and 5 in the committee's statement of task.

Chapter 6 lays out the committee's recommendations and highlights the urgent research needed to understand more fully the role of children in transmission, the risks posed to the community's health by operating schools in person, and the relative effectiveness of the wide range of mitigation strategies that schools are being encouraged to implement.

Discussions related to equity, which is called out in questions 3 and 6 in the statement of task, are threaded throughout the report, and the committee comments on this theme in an Epilogue at the end of this document.

Finally, Appendix A discusses the committee's approach to gathering and reviewing evidence for this study. Appendix B lists the guidance documents reviewed for this report and provides hyperlinks for this guidance as of publication. Appendix C describes a series of examples of how districts are planning to reopen schools, and Appendix D contains biographical sketches of committee members and staff.

2

COVID-19: What Is and Is Not Known

OVID-19 is the name for the clinical disease caused by infection with SARS-CoV-2, a virus first recognized in China in late 2019. COVID-19 is a highly infectious disease that grew rapidly into a major global pandemic resulting in hundreds of thousands of deaths worldwide. This chapter begins with a brief preliminary history of COVID-19. It then reviews current knowledge about the prevalence, distribution, and transmission of COVID-19; its impact on children, adults, and marginalized communities; and preliminary mitigation efforts. The chapter ends with the committee's conclusions on these topics. The committee relied on this science to guide our conclusions and recommendations related to the reopening of K–12 schools later in this report.

PRELIMINARY HISTORY OF COVID-19

The COVID-19 outbreak was first recognized in Wuhan, China, in December 2019. By late January, the World Health Organization (WHO) had declared a public health emergency of international concern on the advice of the agency's emergency committee, marking a global effort to prevent, detect, and respond to the spread of the virus. In the United States, community transmission was first recognized in late February, but likely had been occurring for some time before then. By mid-March, thousands of cases had been identified across the country.

In response to the intense transmission of the virus in the United States, governors took bold steps to curtail the disease, including making unprecedented decisions to close large congregate spaces, such as churches and malls. K–12 schools were among the first institutions to close their buildings, changing access to and modalities of the delivery of education for children. For most school systems, these closures were extended for the rest of the school year and into the summer. As those jurisdictions look ahead to the new school year, they face complex questions about whether and how to reincorporate in-person learning.

As the disease continues to unfold, the committee is reminded of how much has been learned in the past months, yet how much remains to be known to better understand how to construct, operate, and gather in environments in a way that is safe and minimizes the risks to children and their families.

PREVALENCE AND DISTRIBUTION

Globally, as of July 10, 2020, there were more than 12.9 million cases of confirmed COVID-19, with 570,250 deaths attributed to the disease. According to data collated by The Johns Hopkins University, the United States accounts for 135,270 of these deaths as of July 10, 2020.

Of the 3.3 million reported cases in the United States as of July 10, 2020, the Centers for Disease Control and Prevention (CDC) estimates that roughly 5 percent of symptomatic cases in the United States are found among children. However, cases among children are undercounted because of the low volume of COVID-19 testing nationally among the pediatric population, with older age groups and those presenting with severe respiratory symptoms having been the testing priority.

According to the CDC, the vast majority of positive cases are in people aged 18–64. While people under the age of 65 represent a significant number of positive cases, those aged 60–85 who test positive for the virus are at highest risk for severe illness and death. Black, Hispanic[1]/LatinX, and Indigenous populations account for 55 percent of all COVID-19 cases—a disproportionate share given that they represent about 33 percent of the U.S. population.

Not all communities in the United States have been affected by COVID-19 in the same way. States in the Northeast, particularly New York and New Jersey, were hit early and hard, but had begun to turn the corner by mid-April and as of this writing were experiencing relatively low levels of transmission. In contrast, other areas not heavily affected in the first few months of the outbreak, particularly in the South and West, have begun to struggle with increased transmission. These geographic and temporal patterns will likely continue to change as flareups and efforts to regain control

---

[1] The committee uses the term LatinX throughout this report, unless the research cited specifically uses a different term.

change the epidemiological picture. School systems will need to take local epidemiology into account when making decisions about whether and how to open and close.

TRANSMISSION

SARS-CoV-2 is transmitted primarily by respiratory droplets from close contact with infected persons, and by surfaces that have been contaminated by infected persons and then touched by previously uninfected persons who then touch their mouth, nose, or eyes without first properly washing their hands. The average number of secondary cases per infectious case ranges from 2.5 to well over 3.0, making this virus considerably more infectious than influenza (Inglesby, 2020). Current evidence suggests that, given how the virus is spread, prolonged close contact in indoor environments is particularly high risk (Centers for Disease Control and Prevention [CDC], 2020b). The median incubation period, regardless of age, is estimated to be about 5 days, with a range of 2–14 days (Rasmussen and Thompson, 2020).

Scientific knowledge about the impact of the virus on adults and children is evolving. Early studies relying on symptom-based surveillance suggested that children were at lower risk than adults for contracting the disease. According to data through June 18, 2020, just 4.9 percent of confirmed cases in the United States had been diagnosed in children aged 0–17 (CDC, 2020a), a statistic supported by studies showing that the proportion of exposed household members is lower in children than in adults (Jing et al., 2020; Li et al., 2020; Zhang et al., 2020). However, one recent study using contact-based surveillance found that children had been infected at rates similar to those for adults, but that they were either asymptomatic or had symptoms too mild to be detected (Bi et al., 2020). Additional seroprevalence (the level of a pathogen in a population, as measured in blood serum) studies are still needed to understand the prevalence of the disease in children in the United States (Ludvigsson, 2020; Rasmussen and Thompson, 2020).

Although it is clear that onward transmission from infected children is possible, it is not yet clear whether children are less likely to transmit than are adults, on average. Several studies have shown that viral loads in symptomatic children are similar to those of adults. However, studies of viral load do not always correlate well with infectiousness, and little information is available on the infectiousness of asymptomatic or subclinically infected children. These uncertainties make it difficult to evaluate the epidemiological risks of reopening schools. If children are efficient transmitters, evidence from influenza suggests that physically reopening schools (without mitigation measures) could contribute substantially to community spread.

However, if children are not efficient transmitters or if such mitigation measures as use of face coverings are very effective, physically reopening will be safer. See Box 2-1 for a summary of key findings related to transmission.

IMPACT ON CHILDREN

Compared with adults, children who contract COVID-19 are more likely to experience asymptomatic infection or mild upper respiratory symptoms. It is estimated that more than 90 percent of children who test positive for COVID-19 will have mild symptoms, and only a small percentage of symptomatic children (estimates range from 1 to 5 percent) will have severe or critical symptoms (Prather, Wang, and Schooley). Notably, children relative to adults are less likely to develop a fever or cough—two symptoms commonly used to identify cases through symptom-based screening (Lu et al., 2020; U.S. Department of Health and Human Services, 2020). To date, identified risk factors for severe disease among children include age <1 year (and thus not school age) or existing comorbidities. Accordingly, the role of chronic medical conditions in disease severity remains a major concern. A retrospective study of 177 children found that 63 percent of those hospitalized with COVID-19 had underlying conditions, compared with 32 percent of nonhospitalized patients, and 78 percent of critically ill chil-

---

BOX 2-1
Key Findings About Transmission

- The virus is transmitted primarily through exhaled respiratory droplets that contain the virus, though aerosol (very small, floating droplets) transmission and transmission from contaminated surfaces may also play a role.
- When breathing or talking normally, droplets are thought to be capable of traveling about 3-6 feet.
- Sneezing, coughing, singing, loud talking can propel droplets farther.
- Inhaling or ingesting droplets, or getting droplets in your eyes are the main mechanisms of transmission.
- Droplets can land on surfaces and then be transferred to the hands and into the mouth, nose, or eyes. It is unclear how much exposure to the virus through surface contact is necessary to cause an infection.
- Aerosols containing the virus can accumulate in the air in a closed space with limited ventilation such that people can become infected by breathing in virus-containing aerosols.
- The virus does not enter the body through the skin.
- People can be contagious before they show symptoms.
- The role of children in transmission is unclear.

dren had underlying conditions, compared with 57 percent of hospitalized, non–critically ill patients (DeBiasi et al., 2020). In one study summarizing early data from the United States, 77 percent of children hospitalized with COVID-19 had at least one underlying health condition (U.S. Department of Health and Human Services, 2020). In New York City, 8 of 9 (89%) children with severe COVID-19 infection had an underlying condition, compared with 61 percent of children with nonsevere illness (Zachariah et al., 2020).

Recent case reports suggest that a new hyperimmune response known as multisystem inflammatory syndrome (MIS-C) may be a rare sequela of SARS-CoV-2 infection. MIS-C associated with COVID-19 infection has shown moderate to severe impacts on children's vital organs and gastrointestinal and circulatory systems, and according to some evidence has resulted in symptoms similar to those of Kawasaki syndrome, which is characterized by acute inflammation of the blood vessels in children. In Italy, for example, 10 patients with Kawasaki-like disease were identified over the course of 2 months, compared with 19 patients in the preceding 5-year period (Verdoni et al., 2020). In addition, children who have been hospitalized for COVID-19 sometimes require treatment for inflammation of the heart, lungs, kidney, gastrointestinal tract, brain, and eyes. Although the epidemiology of MIS-C has not yet been well characterized, experts suggest that it is rare for COVID-19-positive children to develop the syndrome and that most children diagnosed with MIS-C recover.

There are currently two therapeutics that have received emergency use authorization for treating COVID-19, and researchers around the world are working to develop medicines and vaccines to treat and reduce the virulence of the virus. In the United States, there are more than 457 experimental drugs under development and roughly 144 active clinical trials, according to the U.S. Food and Drug Administration (FDA) (U.S. Food and Drug Administration, 2020). It should be noted that no clinical trials have specifically targeted the treatment of children, and many unanswered questions remain about the best therapeutics for children, in part because of the limited number of cases of symptomatic disease in this population (Castagnoli et al., 2020; Kelvin and Halperin, 2020; Rasmussen and Thompson, 2020).

Population-based data tell only part of the story; how to apply those data to individual children is challenging. While it is clear that children with underlying disease, particularly those with progressive conditions (Bailey et al., 2020), are at increased risk of severe complications, it is not yet known how great the absolute risk of severe COVID-19 disease is for children with more common conditions (e.g., asthma) and how those risks should be counterbalanced against the risks of not attending school. Based on the limited data to date, clear guidelines on which children are at sufficiently high risk to require alternative educational modalities is not possible. Parents need to consult with their child's pediatrician, and accommodations need to be made for children for whom the risk of school attendance is deemed too great.

IMPACT ON ADULTS

Although children make up the majority of school populations, schools are also workplaces for many adults, and decisions around how and when to reopen schools will need to account for risks to these older and at-risk populations as well. Consideration must also be given to household members and other close contacts of children outside of the school setting, some of whom may be vulnerable to severe infection.

COVID-19 infection in adults can cause illness ranging from asymptomatic or mild upper respiratory symptoms to acute respiratory distress. Common symptoms include fever, cough, difficulty breathing, and loss of sense of smell. Severity of illness is associated with age; cumulative rates of hospitalization (as of this writing) range from 27.3 per 100,000 population in adults aged 18–29 to 136 per 100,000 in adults aged 50–64. Those at highest risk of severe illness include people 65 and older and those with underlying health conditions, including chronic lung disease, serious heart conditions, severe obesity, diabetes, chronic kidney disease requiring dialysis, and liver disease, and those who are immunocompromised (CDC, 2020e).

According to the CDC, age-adjusted hospitalization rates are highest among non-Hispanic American Indian or Alaska Native and non-Hispanic Black people, followed by Hispanic or LatinX people. Compared with the non-Hispanic white population, rates of hospitalization are approximately five times higher in the non-Hispanic American Indian or Alaska Native population, 4.5 times higher in the non-Hispanic Black population, and 4 times higher in the Hispanic or LatinX population (CDC, 2020c).

DISPRORTIONATE IMPACTS ON MARGINALIZED COMMUNITIES

Black, LatinX, Native American, immigrant, and marginalized low-income populations have been disproportionately impacted by COVID-19. The rates of exposure, positive tests, and deaths due to complications of the disease are greater among these populations compared with their white counterparts. The CDC reports that age-adjusted hospitalization rates are highest for American Indian or Alaska Native populations at 193.8 per 100,000, followed by non-Hispanic Black (171.8 per 100,000) and Hispanic/LatinX populations (150.3). Asian and white populations have the lowest age-adjusted hospitalization rates, at 44.9 and 37.8 per 100,000, respectively (CCD, 2020c). These statistics vary across the country: in New York City, over 50 percent of tests administered in some communities of color were positive at the height of the outbreak (NYC Department of Health and Mental Hygiene, 2020). These gross disparities not only result in poor clinical outcomes associated with COVID-19 but also include a host of social and financial impacts that further exacerbate the structural challenges experienced by these groups.

There are many emerging explanations as to why people of color have been impacted disproportionately by the disease. One set of explanations relates to health status, such as a higher burden of underlying health conditions and limited access to testing and treatment. However, other factors beyond health status may contribute. For example, people of color and those from other marginalized groups are more likely to be employed in lower-wage jobs that are essential to maintaining the operations and infrastructure of communities—for example, jobs related to building sanitation, food production, transportation, material moving, stock production, and municipal services—and were therefore unable to stay home during shutdowns (Rasmussen and Thompson, 2020). They also are more likely to be unable to quarantine or isolate because of family housing or fear of lost wages due to unpaid sick leave. And they are more likely to be unemployed or to work in multiple part-time jobs, limiting their access to health insurance coverage and ability to pay for medical care.

PRELIMINARY MITIGATION EFFORTS

Efforts undertaken thus far to mitigate the spread of COVID-19 include stay-at-home and shelter-in-place orders; testing and contact tracing; social distancing, hand hygiene, and use of face coverings; personal protective equipment; and temperature screenings.

Stay-at-Home and Shelter-in-Place Orders

Stay-at-home and shelter-in-place orders are emergency measures designed to break chains of transmission and limit the spread of disease by asking or requiring that people remain at home. Beginning in March 2020, schools, businesses, and leisure activities in many states were closed, with only essential businesses and services, such as grocery stores and emergency health care, remaining open. These decisions were made largely by governors at the state level. Although extremely disruptive, these measures were effective at slowing the transmission of COVID-19 to prevent health care systems from becoming overwhelmed and to give public health officials time to improve capacities to expand diagnostic testing and scale contact tracing programs.

Testing and Contact Tracing

Diagnostic testing and contact tracing, also known as case-based management, are outbreak containment strategies that focus specifically on people who are infected and those who have been exposed and are therefore at risk of becoming sick. To implement this strategy, everyone with COVID-19-like symptoms should undergo a diagnostic test and receive the results within, ideally, 24 hours. Those who test positive are asked to remain at home (or in a hospital or hotel, if care or alternative accommodations are needed) for the duration of their illness to avoid exposing others. A public health official contacts the newly diagnosed person and conducts an interview aimed at identifying everyone who was exposed to that individual for 10–15 minutes or more, dating back to 2 days before the onset of symptoms. Public health officials then notify those close contacts about their exposure and ask that they remain at home for 14 days so that should they become ill, they will not expose anyone else. Chains of transmission are thereby broken, and the virus is "boxed in" (Resolve to Save Lives, 2020). Case-based management strategies have allowed a number of countries, including New Zealand, Singapore, and South Korea, to control transmission substantially and safely reopen some community activities.

Physical Distancing, Hand Hygiene

Physical distancing (also called social distancing), hand hygiene, and use of facial coverings are individual-level interventions intended to reduce the risk of infection.

Physical distancing prevents the close contact that makes it easy for the virus to pass from one person to another. Six feet is the most commonly recommended distance in the United States, but this is a rule of thumb, not a definitively safe distance.

Similarly, handwashing reduces the risk of infection from hand-to-face behaviors or during food preparation or other opportunities for the virus to enter the eyes, nose, or mouth. Opportunities for handwashing include before eating; when coming in from outside; after using the bathroom or a facial tissue; and before spending time with others, particularly those at high risk of severe illness. Alcohol-based hand sanitizer may be used if soap and water are not readily available.

Personal Protective Equipment

For health care workers and others in high-risk roles, a higher level of personal protective equipment than that for the general population is recommended to prevent the wearer from becoming infected. The CDC recommends that all health care personnel wear a surgical or procedural face mask at all times while in a health care facility. Personnel caring for someone with a suspected or confirmed case of COVID-19 are recommended to wear an N95 respirator, a face shield or goggles, an isolation gown, and gloves. Additional guidance on personal protective equipment in health care settings is available on the CDC website.[2]

Because of severe supply shortages, medical-grade personal protective equipment is not recommended for use by the general public. The fabric face coverings recommended by the CDC provide only minimal protection to the wearer; they are intended to reduce risk to others. Because one major mode of transmission is through droplets produced during speaking, singing, coughing, or sneezing, facial coverings that act as a barrier to prevent those droplets from spreading can theoretically reduce the risk of transmission. Although this mitigation strategy is not well described in the literature, there is mechanistic plausibility for it, and use of face coverings is now recommended by both the CDC and WHO (World Health Organization, 2019).

Temperature Screenings and Symptom Screenings

Temperature screenings are intended to identify people with a fever that may indicate an infection. The screenings are usually conducted with a noncontact thermometer or according to the CDC's recommended protocol (CDC, 2020b). The effectiveness of temperature screenings as a coronavirus mitigation measure is not known. Although most adults (70%) infected with the virus have a fever at some point in their illness, the proportion is lower for children (Stokes et al., 2020; U.S. Department of Health and Human Services, 2020). In the setting of international travel, temperature screenings have been found to have a low sensitivity (Gostic et al., 2015). In school settings, the CDC recommends that screening be conducted, but it need not be limited to temperature screening; it could also include, for example, symptom screening (CDC, 2020b).

CONCLUSIONS

Conclusion 2.1: Evidence to date suggests that children and youth (aged 18 and younger) are at low risk of serious, long-term consequences or death as a result of contracting COVID-19. Currently, there is insufficient evidence to determine how contagious children and youth are or how likely they are to contract the virus.

---

[2] See https://www.cdc.gov/coronavirus/2019-ncov/hcp/infection-control-recommendations. html.

Conclusion 2.2: Black, LatinX, and Indigenous people; low-income populations; and children and adults with chronic underlying health conditions are disproportionately impacted by COVID-19. Although all people are susceptible to the virus, regardless of race or income, underlying inequities in access to health resources, inflexible employment, and housing and economic issues make certain populations more vulnerable to transmission of and poor outcomes from the disease.

Conclusion 2.3: Mitigation strategies such as physical distancing, hand-washing, use of face coverings, symptom screening, and avoiding large gatherings can reduce the risk of spread of the virus, and will be particularly important in managing how students and adults interact within indoor spaces such as schools and classrooms.

Conclusion 2.4: COVID-19 has more serious health consequences for adults who contract the virus than for children. Mitigation strategies implemented in schools are especially important for protecting school staff and limiting potential transmission of the virus to vulnerable adults in the families of students and school staff.

3

Schools and the Pandemic

In addition to fulfilling the crucial task of educating children, schools serve multiple functions in communities. Many families rely on schools for child care, not only during regular school hours but also through extended care in mornings and after school. Schools also provide meals, health care, counseling, and access to social services. In many communities, moreover, schools serve as a center of social life, a place where everyone gathers for events and where relationships among members of the community are built. Finally, schools are workplaces.

With the closure of schools as a consequence of the COVID-19 pandemic, access to many of these functions was lost. Because of these ripple effects of school closures, communities are wrestling with the difficult question of how best to balance the public health risks involved in opening and operating schools against the consequences for students, families, and communities of keeping them closed. In this chapter we outline the risks of keeping buildings closed and describe aspects of education that are especially relevant to the question of opening and operating school buildings.

THE MULTIPLE PURPOSES OF SCHOOLS

The manifold purposes of schools have never been as evident as they are at this moment, when families are attempting to serve all of those functions at once, at home. Aside from their stated purpose as a place where students are exposed to and learn the academic disciplines, schools fill critical civic and practical roles. Since the "common school" movement of the 1830s, public school advocates have stressed the role of schooling in promoting social cohesion among disparate groups through a universal scholastic experience. In this sense, schools are the quintessential public good: the argument that strong common schooling begets a strong, committed citizenry has long been used to justify why taxpayers should invest in education (Kober and Rentner, 2020).

Schools are also tasked with teaching disciplinary content (such as reading, mathematics, science, etc.), and providing a space where students can develop critically important socioemotional skills. While schools are certainly not the only place students can develop these skills, they are a major venue for children to interact with one another and with adults outside of their families. These interactions in schools provide important opportunities for children and youth to develop self-regulation, essential life skills, and interests and identities.

Schools are also workplaces. In addition to the more than 3.8 million full-time public elementary and secondary teachers employed in schools (McFarland et al., 2019), schools employ leaders and administrators, support staff, maintenance persons, cafeteria workers, nurses and mental health professionals, and others. As a workplace, schools are subject to the same labor laws and health and safety regulations that govern other businesses, and many school employees are represented by labor unions negotiating on their behalf.

On a personal level, families entrust their children to schools with the belief that experienced personnel and staff will act *in loco parentis* by caring for them and keeping them safe from harm. School leaders, educators, and staff play a vital role in ensuring that effective policies, procedures, and strategies are in place to ensure that the physical safety, health and well-being, and nutritional needs of students are met while in their care. Indeed, many schools now serve as a key point of coordination for basic needs supports and community services for some of the nation's most vulnerable students and families. This "child care" function of schools is what enables many parents to participate in the U.S. workforce.

INEQUITY IN AMERICAN EDUCATION

Any discussion of public schools in the United States needs to begin with an acknowledgment of the profound inequities that have characterized the system since it was established. Research shows that schools in which a majority of students come from economically disadvantaged communities often lack the human, material, and curricular resources to meet their students' academic and socioemotional needs (National Academies of Sciences, Engineering, and Medicine [NASEM], 2019a). Relative to their counterparts from wealthier families, students in these under-resourced schools have more limited access to learning opportunities and resources that can promote their success (Owens, Reardon, and Jencks, 2016). This observation is supported by research showing that poverty rates among the families of students who attend a school are associated with key measures of school quality that affect learning and achievement (Bohrnstedt et al., 2015; Clotfelter et al., 2007; Hanushek and Rivkin, 2006). Research also shows that Black and LatinX students are disproportionately more likely to be enrolled in schools with large proportions of low-income students (NASEM, 2019a).

These persistent underlying conditions are a crucial consideration when weighing the costs and benefits of reopening and operating schools during the COVID-19 pandemic. Poorly resourced schools are likely to have fewer resources to devote to developing alternatives to in-person instruction when schools are closed. Low-income students and families are less likely to have access to reliable Internet thus limiting their access to online instruction. Higher-income families may have more resources to devote to enrichment activities than low-income families, and may be more likely to have jobs that allow them to work from home and potentially support children during distance learning. Finally, as we elaborate later in this chapter, the age and condition of school facilities can vary widely even within the same district, creating challenges for implementation of the public health measures neces- sary to limit the spread of COVID-19. Further, schools and school districts vary widely in the funds and staff they can devote to implementing such measures.

In sum, any decision about school reopening and operation has to be informed by existing disparities in resources and infrastructure. Without careful attention to equity and inequity, plans for moving ahead in the 2020–2021 school year run a very real risk of exacerbating the existing inequities in ways that could have serious long-term, detrimental conse- quences for students, families, and communities.

RISKS OF EXTENDED BUILDING CLOSURES

When school buildings closed in Spring 2020, the majority of districts developed strategies for providing distance learning for students. It is likely that if school buildings remain closed for the 2020–2021 school year, dis- tance learning options will be made available. This means that, ultimately, the decision to reopen school buildings entails weighing the potential nega- tive impact of long-term distance learning on children and youth against the health risks of reopening to the community.

Educational Risks to Students

In this section, we discuss the educational risks to children and youth as well as the risks to families and communities if school buildings remain closed. As noted above, schools play an important role in the lives of children and youth not just academically, but also socially, emotionally, and even physically. Impacts in all of these domains need to be considered.

We begin with a brief description of the closures in Spring 2020. We examined the Spring 2020 closures for two reasons. First, they highlight the problem of uneven access when distance learning is the primary mode of instruction. Second, the trends in access suggest that some groups of students may be at greater risk of falling behind academically when distance learning is used for an extended period of time.

Schools' Responses in Spring 2020

In Spring 2020, schools were forced to close quickly with little advance warning and little time to develop robust plans for continuity of instruction or for providing the full range of services outlined above. Nevertheless, district leaders, teachers, and other staff, often alongside parents, went to heroic efforts to continue as many services as possible. A survey of 250 school districts (10,289 schools) nationwide showed that by early May 2020, 97 percent of the districts were providing some kind of distance learning, including both web-based platforms and packets of worksheets (American Enterprise Institute, 2020). Districts varied, however, in the extent to which they provided synchronous instruction (where teachers and students interact virtually in real time) and documented students' participation in learning. Among a representative sample of 477 school systems across the country surveyed following the widespread closures (Gross and Opalka, 2020), only one in three said they expected teachers to provide instruction, track student engagement, or monitor academic progress for all students. Only half of districts expected teachers to track their students' engagement in learning through either attendance tracking or one-on-one check-ins.

The same survey found significant gaps between rural districts and urban and suburban school districts. Only 27 percent of rural and small-town districts expected teachers to provide instruction, compared with more than half of urban districts. Similarly, 43 percent of rural districts expected teachers to take attendance or check in with their students on a regular basis, compared with 65 percent of urban districts. Fewer rural than urban districts required progress monitoring and provided formal grades of some kind. These gaps between rural and urban and suburban districts were larger than the gaps between affluent and economically disadvantaged communities. Still, school districts in affluent communities were twice as likely as those in more economically disadvantaged communities to expect teachers to deliver real-time lessons to groups of students. The variation across districts revealed in these findings raises concern about the disparities in access to instruction that could be created if distance learning were to continue over the long term in the 2020–2021 school year.

Lack of access to the Internet and to devices that facilitate effective virtual learning, as well as limited broadband, also could lead to disparities in access to instruction. According to the American Community Survey, as of 2018, 94 percent of 3- to 18-year-olds had home Internet access: 88 percent had home access through a computer, 6 percent only through a smartphone, and 6 percent not at all. As with other disparities, access varies by socioeconomic status and race/ethnicity. About 26 percent of low-income 3- to 18-year-olds do not have Internet access or have it only through a smartphone, compared with 12 percent of middle low-income families, 5 percent of middle high-income families, and 2 percent of high-income families. Similarly, 30 percent of American Indian or Alaskan Native families do not have access or have it only through a smartphone, as is the case for 24 percent of families of Pacific Islander descent, 21 percent of Black families, 19 percent of LatinX families, 7 percent of white families, and 4 percent of Asian families. Finally, in urban areas, just 2 percent of people lack adequate broadband coverage, compared with 26 percent of those in rural areas and 32 percent of those living on tribal lands (Rachfal and Gilroy, 2019).

Taken together, these trends suggest that low-income students, students of color, and students in rural areas have less access to the technology needed to support virtual learning. Many districts, recognizing these disparities, went to tremendous efforts to improve access by providing devices and hot spots. This may mean that access is less of an issue for the Fall 2020-2021 school year, but the extent to which districts are able to surmount the access issues is likely tied to the amount of resources they have as well as how many students do not have access.

Learning and Instruction in the 2020–2021 School Year

The reality of the current public health situation is that even if school buildings reopen to some extent districts are likely to use a blend of in-person and distance learning. In some locations, the majority of students and teachers may be in the building. However, even where community transmission is minimal and where the school buildings can accommodate all students in new configurations that allow for physical distancing, medically vulnerable students and staff will likely need to have a distance option. This raises the question of how districts should make decisions about how to prioritize which students will be most at risk from extended distance learning and how to ensure that access to distance learning options is equitable.

Children and youth of all ages benefit from in-person learning both academically and socioemotionally. The potential for real-time feedback and discussion, opportunities to interact with peers, and warm, supportive relationships with adults in schools are all key features of in-person learning that are difficult to replicate in distance learning.

The consequences of long-term distance learning are likely to differ depending on the age of students and their specific learning needs. Elementary-aged children may struggle with distance learning, especially if an adult is not available to support them. This is the case especially for children in grades K–3, who are still developing the skills needed to regulate their own behavior and emotions, maintain attention, and monitor their own learning (NASEM, 2019b). As children move into later childhood and adolescence, they become better able to regulate their own emotions and behavior (NASEM, 2019c). In addition, the long-term consequences of being unable to make adequate progress through distance learning may be more severe for students in grades K–3 than for older students. Research has demonstrated long-term, negative consequences for children who are not reading at grade level by third grade, particularly those in low-income families (National Research Council, 1998).

Children and youth with special needs or with individualized education programs may also be at greater risk from long-term distance learning. Even with adequate resources at home, they often cannot derive the same level of service (e.g., career and technical education, physical therapy, medical care) that in-person contact provides.

Finally, as noted in Chapter 2, parents and caregivers who are low-income and are Black, and LatinX are more likely to be employed in jobs where they cannot telecommute. This means that even when students have access to appropriate technology, there may not be an adult in the home during the day who can provide the additional support that some students may need to benefit from distance learning. These trends may mean that long-term use of distance learning can result in even larger disparities in learning outcomes by income and race/ethnicity than already exist.

Recognizing all of these factors, the American Academy of Pediatrics (2020) recently released a statement that "strongly advocates that all policy considerations for the coming school year should start with a goal of having students physically present in school."

Equity and Distance Learning

As noted above, troubling differences exist in access to the Internet and devices that allow students to engage fully in virtual learning. Therefore, a major challenge of developing models for operating schools that include some form of distance learning will be ensuring that all students have equitable access to instruction. Recognizing this challenge, The Education Trust and Digital Promise (2020) collaborated on a guide for digital learning that poses important questions related to equity, identifies key challenges, and offers examples of possible strategies. The key questions are as follows:

1. "How are you ensuring that all students have access to the devices they need to fully participate in distance learning?
2. How are you ensuring that all students have access to reliable, high-speed Internet to continue their education?
3. How are you supporting schools in structuring instructional time to meet the needs of students with varying levels of access to the Internet and technology?
4. How are you supporting students with disabilities who need specialized instruction, related services, and other supports during school closures?
5. How are you ensuring the instructional needs of English Learners are supported during school closures?
6. What kind of support and professional development are you providing to school leaders and teachers, especially in schools serving students of color and students from low-income backgrounds and educators of students with disabilities and English learners?
7. How are you supporting the social and emotional well-being of students, their parents/caregivers, and teachers during school closures?
8. How are you maintaining regular communication with students and families—particularly the most vulnerable—during school closures?
9. How are you measuring student progress to ensure students and families have an accurate picture of student performance for this school year?
10. How are you supporting all high school students, especially seniors, in staying on track to graduate and preparing for college and career?"

Risks to Families and Communities

With the closure of school buildings, districts either stopped providing the various supports and services noted at the beginning of this chapter or had to quickly develop innovative ways of continuing them. Reopening school buildings will allow schools to provide these supports and services more easily and in a more complete way.

Economically disadvantaged children and their families rely on school meals to meet basic nutritional needs. During school closures, school districts were immediately compelled by state and local governments and local education agencies to provide breakfast and lunch to any student, regardless of family income. A survey of 250 public school districts (10,289 schools) showed that although all the schools were closed by late March 2020, 95 percent were providing meals to students as of May 8, 2020 (American Enterprise Institute, 2020). As the COVID-19 pandemic continues to impact economic conditions nationwide, many more families are likely to need access to meals through schools.

In some communities, schools have increasingly become a key point of coordination for health and mental health services for vulnerable students and families. For health services, some schools offer extensive support including health centers located in the school while others offer little support. About 81 percent of public schools employ a full- or part-time school nurse (Willgerodt, Brock, and Maughan, 2018). School nurses conduct screenings, administer medications, address acute injuries and illnesses, and help students get needed care. They also help prevent disease outbreaks by tracking student immunization requirements and monitoring health trends (Willgerodt et al., 2018).

Students and families receive mental health support from a range of professionals in the school setting including school counselors and psychologists. Before being forced by the pandemic to close, many schools were already recognizing the need to provide more extensive mental health supports for students; for some students, schools are the primary source of these supports. Even prior to the pandemic, many children and youth—especially those of low socioeconomic status—experienced traumatic events (Phelps and Sperry, 2020). These adverse events often have long-term negative impacts (Phelps and Sperry, 2020). The pandemic is likely to increase the number of students who need this kind of support, particularly those whose families have experienced economic hardship or death.

If and when schools physically reopen, the socioemotional and mental health needs of students and families will need to be a high priority. While much attention has been paid in the media to potential learning losses and the negative consequences for academic achievement, the collective trauma of the pandemic should not be underestimated. Particularly in the communities hardest hit by COVID-19, children may have experienced the extreme illness or death of multiple close family members even as their families and communities are facing the stress of serious economic setbacks. While it was beyond the scope of the committee's charge to specify how schools should help students and families cope with this trauma, we stress the importance of making this kind of supportive response a priority. These efforts will need to include school counselors and other specialized staff as well as teachers.

Finally, while the time that children and youth spend in school is about much more than child care, public schools do serve as the primary child care option for many working caregivers. The extensive building closures meant that families were left without child care. For caregivers who were able to work from home, this meant juggling work responsibilities while also caring for children and supporting their ongoing learning. However, as noted above, many caregivers, particularly those who are low income, Black, or LatinX, do not have access to jobs that allow them to work from home. Without reliable child care they must make difficult decisions about leaving children home alone, or leaving their jobs.

CONSIDERATIONS FOR OPENING AND OPERATING SCHOOLS DURING COVID-19

While the risks of building closures to students and families discussed above are important to consider, the needs and concerns of the school workforce are equally important. In addition, the condition of school facilities poses practical constraints on how well strategies for maintaining the health of staff and students can be implemented.

The School Workforce

Reopening school buildings safely also means finding a way to ensure the safety of the professionals who work in schools. School districts are often one of the largest employers in local communities. In 2017, elementary, middle, and secondary schools nationwide employed more than 5.5 million people (Bureau of Labor Statistics, 2018). Of these, 3.1 million (65%) were teachers and instructors. Other than teachers, the two largest occupations in schools were janitors and cleaners (300,000) and education administrators (250,000).

Many school personnel are understandably concerned about the health risks involved in returning to full-time, in-person instruction. Twenty-eight percent of public school teachers are over 50, putting them in the higher-risk age category for serious consequences of COVID-19 (Taie and Goldring, 2020). On a survey of teachers, principals, and district leaders administered by the EdWeek Research Center in June 2020, 62 percent reported that they were somewhat or very concerned about returning. Any plans for reopening will need to address these concerns.

The effects of the pandemic on the long-term teacher workforce are still unknown, with some evidence indicating that previous recessions have induced strong candidates to enter the relatively stable teaching profession (Nagler, Piopiunik, and West, 2017). At the same time, many schools, particularly those that serve the least advantaged students, struggled even before the pandemic to fill positions in such areas as upper-level mathematics, science, and special education (Learning Policy Institute, 2018), and there are concerns that reopening schools could exacerbate existing staffing shortages. Just under one-fifth of teachers and almost one-third of principals are aged 55 or older, the age group that accounts for the majority of COVID-19 deaths (Taie and Goldring, 2020; Will, 2020). These are also the teachers who have the option of early retirement, and a wave of concurrent retirements could severely limit schools' options for serving students.

School Facilities and School Organization

The scale of the reopening of U.S. public K–12 school buildings is staggering: prior to the pandemic, nearly 50 million students and 6 million adults attended school in 100,000 buildings, encompassing an estimated 7.5 billion gross square feet and 2 million acres of land (Filardo, 2016). School facility infrastructure was designed to support dense communities of children, managed by adults. Facilities were designed to group students in maximum class sizes; utilize large spaces for eating, outdoor play, and assemblies; and require the sharing of laboratories, art, music, and physical education spaces to reduce costs. The 2017 National Household Travel Survey found that of the 50 million children (aged 5–17) who traveled to school each day in the United States, 54.2 percent were usually driven in a private vehicle, 33.2 percent took a school bus, 10.4 percent walked or biked, and 2.2 percent used other forms of transit (Federal Highway Administration, 2019). At least 35 percent of U.S. schoolchildren travel to school in close proximity to others. School reopening and operating/mitigation strategies will have to be implemented within this organizational structure.

Prior to the pandemic, many students across the country attended school in aging facilities with significant deferred maintenance problems; inadequate cleaning; and obsolete facilities systems, components, and technology. Crowding also characterized many schools and classrooms. Research shows that high-quality facilities help improve student achievement, reduce truancy and suspensions, improve staff satisfaction and retention, and raise property values (Filardo, Vincent, and Sullivan, 2019). They also are integral to ensuring educational equity and opportunities for students and communities (Office of Civil Rights, 2014).

School districts are being advised to employ mitigation measures that are challenging. In order to reopen and operate in the COVID environment, school districts are being advised to monitor and improve their indoor air quality, increase the levels of cleaning, ensure frequent handwashing for students and staff, and employ space utilization to physically distance students and staff. Each of these mitigation measures poses unique operational challenges. They are especially difficult to implement in aged facilities with deferred maintenance and inadequate custodial support.

According to a recently released Government Accountability Office (GAO) report on school facilities, about half (an estimated 54%) of public school districts need to update or replace multiple building systems or features in their schools (U.S. Government Accountability Office, 2020). An estimated 41 percent of districts need to update or replace heating, ventilation, and air conditioning (HVAC) systems in at least half of their schools, representing about 36,000 schools nationwide. Ventilation and air filtration are among the mitigation measures schools are asked to consider. These measures include taking steps to increase the amount of fresh air in classrooms and other occupied areas, installing HEPA filters in mechanical systems, and moving instruction outdoors. Schools with modern HVAC systems are able to implement the HVAC mitigation recommendations; as the GAO study shows, however, this is not the case for nearly half of the nation's public schools.

Many school districts, particularly those serving low-income students, already suffer from having inadequate custodial staff. Cleaning to higher standards will require hiring and training additional custodial staff and procuring additional cleaning supplies and equipment. Older school facilities will not have enough bathrooms or sinks for frequent handwashing. The faucets and fixtures of lavatories that are in poor condition will not be in full working order, making frequent handwashing protocols difficult to implement.

Staffing schools to meet the Centers for Disease Control and Prevention's (CDC's) physical distancing guideline of a minimum 6-foot separation between students is also a major challenge for districts. Class sizes currently vary tremendously. Children with high levels of needs, including those who are medically fragile, are in very small groups of as few as 6 students, while typical class sizes are anywhere from 18 to 35 students, depending on age, subject, and the resources of the school district. Physical distancing with class size limited to as few as 10–18 students per class, depending on classroom square footage, will require more instructional staff. School districts are exploring major schedule changes to meet the CDC's physical distancing guideline, with students spending far less time in onsite instruction. Meeting that guideline is even more challenging for poorly resourced districts. Insufficient in-school technology infrastructure, for example, means that synchronous instruction that could serve students both onsite and offsite will be difficult if not impossible.

Many studies have found that poor-quality school facilities harm occupant health, attendance, achievement, and school quality,[1] and children

---

[1] There is strong evidence in the academic literature that the quality of school facilities affects student achievement through myriad factors, and is a factor in student and teacher attendance, teacher retention and recruitment, child and teacher health, and the quality of curriculum (Alexander and Lewis, 2014). Researchers at the Harvard School of Public Health recently wrote, "the evidence is unambiguous—school buildings impact student health, thinking, and performance" (Allen et al., 2017, p. 3). Poor or substandard school buildings and grounds negatively affect the health of children and adults in schools, which in turn negatively affects

from low-income and nonwhite communities disproportionately attend schools with such facilities (Filardo et al., 2006). These conditions complicate reopening decisions and COVID-19 mitigation strategies (Filardo, 2016).

CONCLUSIONS

Conclusion 3.1: Keeping schools closed to in-person learning in Fall 2020 poses potential educational risks for all students. Children and youth benefit from learning experiences that include support from a teacher and interactions with peers. Even when it includes virtual interactions, distance learning cannot take the place of in-person interaction. Young relative to older children and youth are less able to engage effectively in distance learning without adult support. Additionally, it is often more difficult to provide a robust educational experience for students with disabilities in distance learning settings. As a result, the educational risks of long-term distance learning may be higher for young children and children with disabilities.

Conclusion 3.2: Opening school buildings/campuses for in-person learning to some extent in Fall 2020 would provide benefits for families beyond educating children and youth. Working caregivers would have affordable, reliable child care for school-age children, and families would be better able to access services offered through the school, such as provision of meals and other family supports (e.g., mental health services, school-based health services).

Conclusion 3.3: Even if schools open for some in-person learning in Fall 2020, they are likely to need to continue providing some distance learning for a subset of students. However, schools and communities vary in whether they have the infrastructure necessary to provide high-quality virtual learning for all children and youth. Without careful implementation, virtual learning alone runs the risk of exacerbating existing disparities in access to high-quality education across different demographic groups and communities.

---

their performance (Uline and Tschannen-Moran, 2008). Studies also have found significant correlations between poor structural, conditional, and aesthetic attributes of school buildings and low student learning and achievement (Maxwell, 2016). Likewise, most, though not all, studies examining the relationship between school facility investments and student achievement have found a relationship (see, e.g., Cellini, Ferreira, and Rothstein, 2010; Conlin and Thompson, 2017; Martorell, Stange, and McFarlin, 2016; and Neilson and Zimmerman, 2014).

Conclusion 3.4: Staffing is likely to be a major challenge if schools reopen for in-person instruction in Fall 2020. A significant portion of school staff are in high-risk age groups or are reluctant to return to in-person schooling because of the health risks. In addition, some of the strategies for limiting the transmission of COVID-19 within schools, such as maintaining smaller class sizes and delivering both in-person and virtual learning, will require additional instructional staff.

Conclusion 3.5: Children and youth from low-income families dispro-portionately attend schools with poor-quality facilities. Poor-quality school buildings (i.e., those that have bad indoor air quality, are not clean, or have inadequate bathroom facilities) complicate reopening while the COVID-19 pandemic continues and make it difficult for school districts to implement the recommended health and safety mea-sures. Physically reopening schools with poor-quality school buildings that hinder mitigation measures may make reopening during the pan-demic riskier for occupants.

4

Deciding to Reopen Schools

As stated in Chapter 1, decisions around how to reopen schools are among the most complex and consequential of the COVID-19 pandemic. In this chapter, the committee considers the available epidemiological evidence as well as the needs and priorities of U.S. education stakeholders to offer guidance on these decisions. The discussion in this chapter responds to questions 1 and 3 in the committee's statement of task (see Box 1-1). Taking what is known about decision-making in this moment together with principles from existing guidance documents, we offer a path forward for decision-makers in establishing a clear plan for reopening schools that is based on shared goals and values, ongoing risk assessment, and careful context monitoring.

UNDERSTANDING RISK AND
DECISION-MAKING DURING COVID-19

A 1996 National Academies report entitled *Understanding Risk: Informing Decisions in a Democratic Society* suggests that risk characterization

> must be seen as an integral part of the entire process of risk decision-making: what is needed for successful characterization of risk must be considered at the very beginning of the process and must to a great extent drive risk analysis. If a risk characterization is to fulfill its purpose, it must (1) be decision driven, (2) recognize all significant concerns, (3) reflect both analysis and deliberation, with appropriate input from the interested and

affected parties, and (4) be appropriate to the decision (National Research Council, 1996, p. 16).

From the outset of this work, the committee has acknowledged the tremendous challenges associated with characterizing risk such that stakeholders can make cogent, safe decisions around reopening schools in the time of COVID-19. Among other things, decision-makers must weigh competing priorities that include the pressures of different constituent groups, the need to reopen schools to facilitate parents' full-time return to the workforce, beliefs and perceptions around the import of school for students' socioemotional and academic well-being, labor demands from every type of staff person working in schools, looming fiscal constraints, and the health and safety concerns of parents.

Beyond this complex set of priorities, the committee recognizes the tremendous physical and emotional strains faced by all stakeholders in the education system: as of this writing, the majority of schools in the United States had been closed for in-person learning since March 2020, and a large swath of parents had been without child care. Beyond having to engage with state and local virus mitigation strategies (e.g., stay-at-home orders, mandated use of face coverings) and witnessing the tremendous loss of life experienced by many communities, critical stakeholders face the very real threat of "decision fatigue."[1] The committee also recognizes that many communities of color have joined together to lead historic protests toward advancing racial justice in the United States, and concerns about reopening schools will necessarily take place against that backdrop.

The public health risk from COVID-19 *is* the reason that schools closed in Spring 2020. As the start of the 2020–2021 school year approaches and districts and schools contemplate reopening for in-person activities (whether fully or partially) it is important to understand that it will not be possible to prevent transmission entirely. The increased contact that will occur when people come together in the school, even with many mitigation measures in place, will more than likely lead to new cases of the virus. The question is not a matter of whether there will be cases of SARS-CoV-2 in schools, but what the spread of the virus will look like once cases begin to emerge. Stakeholders need to understand this risk and be willing to move forward with reopening for in-person learning despite it.

In light of this complex constellation of considerations, the committee notes that decisions about reopening schools are likely to be more iterative and ongoing. As circumstances change and understanding of COVID-19

---

[1] Decision fatigue is the idea that the act of making choices repeatedly can lead to depletion of the decider's psychological resources, which can lead to less optimal choosing over time (Vohs et al., 2008).

grows, states, districts, and schools will likely need to decide and redecide not only whether to reopen but also how to know when it may be necessary to shut down again. Later in this chapter, we outline a framework for advancing that iterative decision-making by relevant stakeholders in a given community.

EXISTING GUIDANCE FOR SCHOOLS

As part of its charge, the committee reviewed the rapidly emerging guidance documents related to reopening K–12 schools. While a robust analysis of the content of these documents is beyond the scope of our charge (see Box 1-1 in Chapter 1), we did note a few themes in this guidance related to who should make decisions about reopening schools and how best to make those decisions.

One important issue the committee identified—one also highlighted by a number of presenters during the committee's information-gathering sessions—is that the majority of state-level guidance documents do not explicitly call on districts to reopen schools, but are framed as a series of questions for districts to ask while making decisions about reopening. While this approach to providing guidance does allow for regional variation and sensitivity to contextual factors, it also leaves school districts with a tremendous responsibility for determining how to meet their obligations to students, families, and staff. Many school districts are left without a clear roadmap for understanding just what kind of schooling they are responsible for as the pandemic continues with respect to both academic experiences and the many social services schools are required to provide (see Chapter 3). In addition, placing the full burden on districts leaves open the possibility that if a student, a staff person, or someone in the community contracts COVID-19 in the school, the district will be held responsible.

Guidance provided by the Centers for Disease Control and Prevention (CDC)—in particular, the "decision tree" included with its formal guidance—serves as the basis for most state-level documents on school reopening. A challenge of the CDC decision tree is that it states that hygiene, cleaning, and physical distancing should be implemented "as feasible." Districts are left to make judgment calls about the extent to which they should push to implement all of the recommended strategies and what the consequences might be of relaxing one or the other of those strategies. Some districts may have ready access to experts in infectious disease and public health who can provide input for these decisions, but others do not. For example, many rural communities have either a small or no local health department, and personnel in those agencies may have limited expertise in infectious diseases (Cheney, 2020; Eisenhauer and Meit, 2016).

A close, ongoing partnership between education leaders and departments of public health that starts during planning for reopening is essential.

Such a partnership is particularly important for continuing to monitor the incidence of COVID-19 in schools. The need for this partnership, however, raises the question of how communities where both the schools and the public health infrastructure are under-resourced will be able to maintain the health of the community when schools reopen.

In looking across the guidance documents, the committee felt it was especially important to point out the challenging reality facing school districts that are now responsible for making the majority of decisions related to school reopening. As noted above, this local decision-making is reasonable insofar as it accounts for the significant variation in the spread and prevalence of COVID-19 across different parts of a given state. Further, districts differ in their goals for schooling; as we discuss below, districts across a state are likely to have different supports in place for distance learning models. Different communities in the same state will inevitably have different kinds of needs associated with in-person education. That said, Chapter 3 describes the reality that districts within the same state are likely to have significantly different resources (financial, human capital, etc.) to put toward reopening schools. In light of the fiscal challenges many school districts will face in the 2020–2021 school year, states will need to have a role in ensuring an equitable distribution of resources and expertise so that districts can implement the measures required for a strategic reopening in their local contexts.

A FRAMEWORK FOR DECIDING WHEN TO REOPEN SCHOOLS FOR IN-PERSON LEARNING

Given the range of stakeholders invested in decisions around reopening schools, the committee recognizes that those decisions and processes will be complex. In most cases, decisions about reopening are within the purview of the district superintendent and school board. In this context of multiple stakeholders and often conflicting priorities, the committee recognized that a data-driven, real-time decision-making framework can help stakeholders break down the decision-making process into manageable, informed steps.

To articulate such a framework, the committee turned to testimony provided as part of our information-gathering process by epidemiologist and professor of integrative biology Dr. Lauren Ancel-Meyers of the University of Texas. The University of Texas COVID-19 Modeling Consortium Framework (Box 4-1) can be used in pursuit of three main objectives: (1) help decision-makers establish goals for reopening and the levels of risk they are willing to assume in pursuit of those goals, (2) determine what policy and mitigation strategies are reasonable and desirable, and (3) establish a protocol for continuous feedback through data monitoring.

BOX 4-1

**University of Texas COVID-19 Modeling Consortium
Framework for Decision-Making on Reopening Schools**

What are the goals and constraints? Examples include
- Educational and service objectives
  - o For example, Is the goal to maximize in-person school days? Ensure education by any modality? Meet other health, resource, and safety needs?
- Mitigate COVID-19 risks
  - o Recognize that a zero-tolerance policy may not be feasible
  - o Determine acceptable levels of risk, numbers of cases, absenteeism, etc.

What are the policy and structural options? Examples include
- Establish masks, hygiene, and distancing measures; set facility capabilities; identify priority groups for on-campus activities
- Special precautions for high-risk groups (e.g., cocooning)
- School closures of various durations
- Rapid testing, tracing, and isolation to contain clusters
- Organize various measures into clear stages

How exactly should risk be tracked and used to drive policy? Examples include
- Understand and monitor the available data
  - o Confirmed cases, hospitalizations, deaths in schools or community, absenteeism, health screening in person or via app, etc.
- Set clear thresholds for enacting or relaxing measures

SOURCE: Dr. Lauren Ancel-Meyers, expert testimony to the committee.

The University of Texas COVID-19 Modeling Consortium Framework, although not specifically developed for school reopening decisions, supports education stakeholders in working with public health officials to continually make and remake decisions based on data as they become available (for more information on who should make these decisions, see the following section). The steps in the decision-making process, outlined in Box 4-1, are described below.

First, the framework directs decision-makers to establish values, goals, and priorities for reopening schools. For example, does a community want students to attend school in person because parents are in overwhelming need of child care? Or are stakeholders determined to ensure continuity of learning by any available means, including virtual or distance learning modalities? Ancel-Meyers suggests that once those goals have been established, decision-makers can weigh the goals against the level of risk they are willing to assume: What is the threshold of case counts this community is willing to accept before closing in-person facilities? What levels of absenteeism are acceptable to keep a majority of students in classrooms?

In step 2, stakeholders and decision-makers review mitigation strategies and policy options for schools. It is at this point in the process that stakeholders will need to be explicit about what the constraints are on the various policy options on the table: for example, schools and districts may need to conduct an assessment of how robust the current distance learning infrastructure is for supporting at-home learning. Stakeholders may also want to consider local variability in seasons as they make plans to support fresh air exchange in classrooms, or even consider whether outdoor learning is a realistic possibility.

Finally, stakeholders will need to establish protocols for collecting and monitoring data related to the COVID-19 context in the community. In this process, relevant decision-makers establish clear thresholds for what those data mean; for example, once a school sees X number of cases, it will enact Y policy. Figure 4-1 illustrates how the city of Austin, Texas, is operationalizing this staged approach to reopening schools and businesses.

In the case of Austin, Texas, thresholds for the staging of community reopening are determined by using the number of 7-day average hospital admissions to understand the level of ongoing risk posed by COVID-19. In the red stage (more than 70 long-term hospital admissions), the city is open only to essential businesses, and mitigation strategies for all individuals (masks, physical distancing) are in place, regardless of their personal risk status. As case counts decline, the city moves from Stage 5 down to Stage 1. As the city proceeds through stages, mitigation strategies slowly ease—first for lower-risk individuals and then for higher-risk individuals—and more businesses open up. If case counts increase, the city can move back to an earlier stage of intervention, depending on the level of COVID-19 risk.

The state of Oregon is using a similar approach for the reopening of schools and businesses (https://govstatus.egov.com/reopening-oregon#baseline), with counties submitting plans and data to the state to receive approval for moving through different phases of reopening. Counties must demonstrate progress on seven indicators: declining prevalence of COVID-19, minimum testing requirements, clear and actionable plans for contact tracing, identified locations for safe isolation and quarantine, a clear plan for keeping workers safe and healthy, sufficient health care capacity, and a sufficient supply of personal protective equipment. As progress on these indicators is demonstrated, restrictions on businesses and individual behaviors ease.

Districts, local health officials, and communities could operationalize similar approaches in establishing plans for reopening schools that leverage potential mitigation strategies and policies together with ongoing data monitoring. Chapter 5 details the mechanisms that need to be in place to

COVID-19: Risk-Based Guidelines

Recommended thresholds / 7-day average hospital admits	Stage	Practice Good Hygiene (Stay Home If Sick / Avoid Sick People)	Maintain Social Distancing	Wear Facial Coverings	Higher Risk Individuals Aged 65+, diabetes, high blood pressure, heart, lung and kidney disease, immunocompromised, obesity			Avoid Gatherings	Avoid Non-Essential Travel	Avoid Dining/Shopping	Workplaces Open
					Avoid Gatherings	Avoid Non-Essential Travel	Avoid Dining/Shopping				
0	Stage 1	•			Greater than 25		Except with precautions	Gathering size TBD			All businesses
< 10	Stage 2	•	•	•	Greater than 10		Except as essential	Greater than 25			Essential and reopened businesses
10 - 39	Stage 3	•	•	•	Social and greater than 10	•	Except as essential	Social and greater than 10			Essential and reopened businesses
40 - (70 to 123)*	Stage 4	•	•	•	Social and greater than 2	•	Except as essential	Social and Greater than 10	•	Except expanded essential businesses	Expanded essential businesses
> (70 - 123)* (depending on rate of increase)	Stage 5	•	•	•	Outside of household	•	Except as essential	Outside of household	•	Except as essential	Essential businesses only

* The exact hospitalization average trigger will depend on the rate of increase. A faster increase in the daily average will trigger stage 5 risk recommendations when the number reaches the lower end of this range.

Use this color-coded alert system to understand the stages of risk. This chart provides recommendations on what people should do to stay safe during the pandemic. Individual risk categories identified pertain to known risks of complication and death from COVID-19. This chart is subject to change as the situation evolves.

AustinTexas.gov/COVID19   Published: June 26, 2020   APH Austin Public Health

FIGURE 4-1 Austin-Travis County COVID-19 risk-based guidelines.
SOURCE: austintexas.gov/COVID19.

ensure that states, districts, and schools can carry these plans forward in implementing the reopening of schools, and Appendix C provides a number of examples for how districts are planning to reopen in Fall 2020.

APPROACHES TO COLLECTIVE DECISION-MAKING

As a process for deciding whether schools should reopen is established, schools and districts will need to ensure that the decisions made reflect their community's priorities. To this end, school districts and communities must be willing to listen and co-plan with community members in order to engage all relevant constituent groups.

In May 2020, the Southern Regional Education Board (SREB) released a "playbook" for enhancing or establishing a local task force to address issues related to COVID-19. This document describes in depth both what kinds of stakeholders should be involved in decision-making (see Box 4-2) and a series of five action items that the task force should take up (discussed later in this chapter). After reviewing this document and considering expert

BOX 4-2
Suggested Members of a School
District's COVID-19 Task Force

State and District	Schools	Other Representatives
• Board of education members • Legislators • Superintendent • Assessment director • Chief academic officer • Communications director • Curriculum and instruction director • Exceptional student • services director • Finance director • Federal grants coordinator • Facilities director • Food and nutrition director • Human resources director • Operations director • Policy director • School safety director • Support services director • Technology director • Transportation director	• Administrators • Teachers • Parents • Students • Community members • School nurses, or school-based health care providers*	• Associations for teachers, school boards, superintendents and principals • The state community college system and higher education agency • Child care agencies or providers • Public television stations • State or local public health departments • Hospitals or health care providers • Mental health officials or clinicians • Public safety agencies • County emergency management • Telecommunication networks • Workforce development agencies • Business partners • Representatives from relevant labor unions*

*Indicates category added by the committee.
SOURCE: © 2020 Southern Regional Education Board. Used with permission.

testimony provided as part of our information-gathering process, the committee agrees that community engagement in decisions related to reopening can help ensure that the divergent concerns of education stakeholders are, at a minimum, brought to light and taken into account. In the absence of this kind of community input, decision-makers risk the possibility that school staff and families will not understand the values or logic behind certain choices, potentially leading some stakeholders to divest from schools altogether.

In particular, districts can deepen partnerships with families and communities by involving them in planning for the reopening of schools; the decision to reopen; the preparation of students for learning; and implementation of newly required policies, procedures, and plans. This involvement is particularly important for families and communities historically marginalized by public systems, which often experience the greatest impact from inequitable schooling.

The SREB (2020) report identifies five major action items for a community task force once it has been assembled:

1. Define the problem the task force will address, and establish a clear scope and purpose to guide the group's work.
2. Define a timeline for the work of the task force, and communicate it to task force members and other shareholders.
3. Identify and secure the participation of task force members, ensuring that the membership is balanced and aligns with the group's communicated purpose.
4. Gather background information and secure available resources.
5. Establish a multifaceted communication plan.

Attending to these items up front makes it possible to then focus on the actual work of making decisions related to reopening schools.

The committee notes that while the precise details of both who is involved in the planning processes and the processes themselves are likely to change depending on local needs, an inclusive process whereby stakeholders are asked to be explicit about their goals, values, and priorities will yield long-term benefits when challenging real-time decisions must be made. The committee also notes that a truly inclusive process for decision-making is not merely about ensuring diverse perspectives at the table, but also about conversations designed such that multiple parties can truly engage. Task forces may want to consider providing supports for families with first languages other than English to ensure that their voices, priorities, and interests are included in the decision-making process. Task forces may also want to leverage partnerships with community organizations to help in assessing the comfort of families with returning to school, as well as in making information accessible to diverse families through such communication strategies as live-streamed meetings and public (socially distanced) town halls.

Additionally, task forces need to consider transparent communication of the reality that while measures can be implemented to lower the risk of transmitting COVID-19 when schools reopen, there is no way to eliminate that risk entirely. It is critical to share both the risks and rewards of different scenarios, and to consider interventions that can be implemented to communicate to families that every effort is being made to keep their children safe in schools. While all stakeholders will not necessarily agree with the final decisions about when and how to reopen schools, an inclusive process will help build trust in school leadership so that decisions can be implemented quickly should conditions change.

MONITORING COVID-19 CONDITIONS

Schools and districts will need to work with their state or local health departments to plan for the monitoring and evaluation of epidemiological data to iteratively assess disease activity in the county (or relevant area). Indicators of particular interest include the number of new cases diagnosed, the number of new hospitalizations and deaths, and the percentage of diagnostic tests that are positive. Schools also will need to monitor absenteeism and alert public health officials to any large increases (Centers for Disease Control and Prevention [CDC], 2020a). According to the CDC's school decision tree, communities with substantial community transmission may need to implement extended school closures. For this reason, the committee notes that it is especially important that decisions about what constitutes substantial community transmission and under what conditions schools would again close will need to be outlined *before* the school year begins. Finally, stakeholders tasked with monitoring data may also want to consider how to ensure that the data are disaggregated by race, class, and (depending on the size of the school or district) zip code. Given what is known about the disproportionate impacts of COVID-19 on under-resourced communities, disaggregated data may offer targeted insight into how to approach mitigation equitably.

One particularly effective strategy for monitoring COVID-19 conditions is to implement a testing program that assists in screening for positive cases. Currently, the CDC recommends that schools refer the following individuals to health care officials for further evaluation: (a) individuals with signs or symptoms consistent with COVID-19, and (b) asymptomatic individuals with recent known or suspected exposure to SARS-CoV-2 to control transmission. School staff are not currently expected to perform tests themselves, although they may serve that purpose in their capacity in school-based health care centers. Finally, the CDC does *not* recommend universal testing of students and staff (i.e., testing everyone even if asymptomatic), because it is not currently understood whether or not a universal testing program contributes to a reduction in transmission (CDC, 2020c). Further, as the CDC guidance on testing and tracing notes,

> Implementation of a universal approach to testing in schools may pose challenges, such as the lack of infrastructure to support routine testing and follow up in the school setting, unknown acceptability of this testing approach among students, parents, and staff, lack of dedicated resources, practical considerations related to testing minors and potential disruption in the educational environment (CDC, 2020c).

To the extent that testing is part of a school's monitoring plan, it may consider partnering with a local health department to implement a contact tracing program. Contract tracing involves identifying individuals who come into contact with others who have tested positive for COVID-19, and asking affected individuals to voluntarily quarantine for 2 weeks to curtail transmission. Although the combination of robust testing and contact tracing programs can serve as a useful strategy in limiting transmission, it may require a substantial investment of local resources. As we discuss in detail in Chapter 5 of this report, schools and districts will need to the weigh the benefits of testing and tracing against the costs and utility of the numerous other mitigation strategies that will need attention.

Monitoring will need to occur at the individual level as well. All staff and parents of children should have initial and periodic training on basic infectious disease precautions, including the identification and management of symptomatic personnel and students, and instructions to remain at home if symptoms do appear. The CDC has guidance for parents (CDC, 2020b).

CONCLUSIONS

Conclusion 4.1: Decisions to reopen schools for in-person instruction and to keep them open have implications for multiple stakeholders in communities. These decisions require weighing the public health risks against the educational risks and other risks to the community. This kind of risk assessment requires expertise in public health, infectious disease, and education as well as a clear articulation of the values and priorities of the community.

Conclusion 4.2: A decision-making framework *and* an inclusive process for making decisions can help support community trust in school and district leadership so that decisions can be implemented quickly throughout the school year.

Conclusion 4.3: Education leaders need to have a way to monitor data on the virus so they can track community spread. If there is substantial community spread, schools may need to close for in-person learning. Decisions about what constitutes substantial community transmission and under what conditions schools would again close need to be outlined before the school year begins.

5

Reducing Transmission When School Buildings Are Open

The decision to reopen school buildings also involves developing a plan for how schools will operate once they are open and how to balance minimizing risk to students and staff while being realistic about cost and practicality. It is important to bear in mind that in order to protect the health of staff, students, their families, and the community, schools will not be able to operate "as normal."

This chapter addresses areas that districts must consider when they are developing plans for reopening: implantation of mitigation strategies, creating a culture for maintaining health, and what to do if someone in the building tests positive for the virus. We begin with an overview of the "hierarchy of controls," a framework for approaching environmental safety in workplaces that is useful for organizing implementation plans. This is followed by a discussion of the most common mitigation strategies for reducing the transmission of COVID-19 in light of existing epidemiological data, published guidance from the Centers for Disease Control and Prevention (CDC), and practicality in school settings. We then provide brief commentary on what to do when someone tests positive. The chapter ends with the committee's conclusion with respect to mitigation strategies for schools. This chapter responds to questions 2, 3, 4, and 5 in the statement of task (see Box 1-1).

It is important to emphasize that this chapter is not meant to replace the guidance issued by the CDC or by states. Rather, the committee offers considerations intended to help districts think through their implementation plans based on the scientific community's understanding of transmission of the SARS-CoV-2 virus as of July 6, 2020. In addition, the committee does not discuss the steps needed to safely reopen buildings that have been closed for a long period of time (e.g., the safety of the water or heating, ventilation, and air conditioning [HVAC] systems). Districts should follow guidance on this provided by the CDC.

IMPLEMENTING MITIGATION STRATEGIES

As discussed in Chapter 2, and noted in the CDC guidance, COVID-19 is mostly spread by respiratory droplets released when people breathe, talk, cough, or sneeze. The virus may also spread to the hands from a contaminated surface and then to the nose, mouth, or eyes, causing infection. This means strategies that limit spread of and exposure to the droplets are the most important for mitigating transmission. As the CDC notes, the risk of transmission in schools is highest when there are "full sized, in-person classes, activities, and events. Students are not spaced apart, share classroom materials or supplies, and mix between classes and activities." Risk is lowered when "groups of students stay together and with the same teacher throughout/across school days and groups do not mix. Students remain at least 6 feet apart and do not share objects."

The guidance provided by the CDC identifies numerous strategies that can be implemented in school to lower risk of transmission. Implementing the full set of strategies may be difficult in many districts due to costs, practical constraints, and the condition of school buildings. As noted in Chapter 4, the decision tree provided by the CDC recognizes these constraints in saying that strategies be implemented "as feasible." While this gives districts flexibility in developing their plans, it also leaves district leaders with the challenge of making judgment calls about how much they should push to implement all of the recommended strategies and what the consequences might be of relaxing some of the strategies.

The major challenge for everyone trying to make judgments about the effectiveness of the various strategies in schools is that the evidence about COVID-19 is still emerging. As a result, the committee was not able to provide strong, definitive guidance on the relative effectiveness of each of the various strategies schools are considering to limit the spread of the virus. However, the committee does offer commentary on the strategies that are especially important to implement well based on current understanding of the disease and lessons learned from research on other viruses.

In this section, the committee identifies a set of key mitigation strategies that schools could implement to reduce the spread of the virus that causes COVID-19. To develop this set of strategies, the committee referred to the CDC guidance for schools as well as guidance from states in conjunction with committee members' understanding of evidence about transmission. In addition, the committee heard expert testimony from epidemiologists and infectious disease doctors who offered their perspectives on which strategies are most promising and which are less likely to be effective (for more information on this process, see Appendix A). We also considered existing infrastructure in schools and additional cost to implement.

The Hierarchy of Controls

To organize the discussion of strategies, the committee used the hierarchy of controls framework. The hierarchy of controls, an approach to environmental safety, is a framework used in many workplaces to prioritize strategies for minimizing people's exposure to environmental hazards (Figure 5-1). This hierarchy structures protective measures according to five levels:

1. Elimination
2. Substitution
3. Engineering
4. Administrative
5. Personal Protective Equipment (PPE)

Generally, strategies that fall within the levels at the top of the hierarchy are viewed as more effective than those within the levels at the bottom.

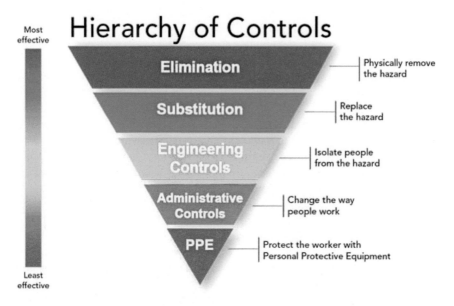

FIGURE 5-1 The Hierarchy of Controls.
SOURCE: National Institute for Occupational Safety and Health, 2015.

This means that when this framework is used, the top levels—elimination, substitution, and engineering controls—are given higher priority. In the context of an infectious disease, however, which strategies need to be prioritized at each level is determined by the route of transmission of the disease. A disease that is spread only by direct physical contact requires different engineering or administrative controls relative to a disease that is spread through droplets. The challenge in the case of the current pandemic is that the transmission of COVID-19, particularly the role of children in transmission, is still not entirely understood (see Chapter 2).

Applying the hierarchy of controls to COVID-19 and schools, elimination and substitution do not apply to school buildings as they reopen. Elimination would be complete control of the virus or a widely distributed vaccine. Substitution means replacing a hazard (in this case the virus) or a hazardous way of operating (being in school) with a nonhazardous or less hazardous substitute. Since COVID-19 cannot be "replaced," the option here is to adopt new, safer processes—for example, moving to distance learning. As discussed in Chapter 3, however, this option may have negative consequences for children, families, and communities if implemented for long periods of time.

Engineering controls eliminate a hazard before an individual comes into contact with it. In the case of COVID-19, such strategies could include improving ventilation, erecting barriers around an area (for example, for front office staff), changing the configurations of classrooms to allow for physical distancing, and performing regular cleaning.

Administrative controls change the way people work. In the context of schools, this means eliminating large gatherings, creating groupings of students and patterns of movement that limit contact with other people, instituting handwashing routines, emphasizing coughing and sneezing etiquette, and providing training in the new routines. The majority of the CDC guidelines fall into this category of controls. Finally, PPE, masks and face shields, is lowest in the hierarchy of controls.

The best way to manage the risk of viral spread in schools is to implement strategies at all three levels (engineering, administrative, and PPE). Given the current context, however, with only an emerging understanding of transmission and how it relates to children, it is difficult to provide evidence-based guidance as to which specific strategies at each level will be most effective. One potential pitfall of implementing strategies based strictly on the hierarchy of controls is that doing so could drive schools to focus primarily on implementing all possible strategies at the engineering level first, on the assumption that this is the most effective way to limit exposure. However, the emerging evidence about COVID-19 suggests that several strategies at the administrative level—including creating routines that allow for physical distancing, eliminating large gatherings, and stressing handwashing—are very important for limiting transmission (see Chapter 2 for more discussion of transmission). In addition, there is increasing evidence that wearing masks can lower transmission. The following section highlights strategies that appear to be especially important to implement or that receive substantial attention in districts' plans (see Table 5-1 for a summary of the strategies).

Personal Protective Equipment

Ideally, all students and staff, including elementary children, should wear fabric face coverings or surgical masks. For teachers and staff, N95 masks would be most effective, but would be difficult to teach in. Surgical masks offer better protection than cloth masks, but may not be available. Requiring only staff to wear masks is less effective because the fabric face coverings recommended by the CDC do not fully protect the wearer from droplets. Rather, the masks are most effective for reducing spread from people who are infected by containing droplets. Children in early elementary grades, especially kindergartners, may have difficulty complying with mask usage. Nonetheless, efforts should be made to encourage compliance. (Strategies for encouraging mask use and other new health behaviors are discussed in a later section.)

Face shields have been recommended by some researchers as an alternative to face masks, and may be an option that would allow students to see teachers' faces (Perencevich, Diekema, and Edmond, 2020). However, the relative effectiveness of using face shields in lieu of fabric masks is unknown, and neither the CDC nor the World Health Organization has commented on this as an option for control of SARS-CoV-2 in the community. Considering that face shields allow droplets and aerosols to escape into the surrounding air, it is unlikely that face shields alone can be as effective as other types of masks.

Implementing all of the COVID spread mitigation strategies fully and faithfully will maximize protection of students and staff. However, districts and schools have limits on staff, time, and resources. Additionally, each school and school community will have unique qualities and the public health conditions in communities will vary. Table 5-1 is provided for stakeholders and districts to use to evaluate how to apply mitigation strategies in their schools given the limits to their resources and what is now known about the mechanics of how these mitigation strategies affect the spread of the virus.

TABLE 5-1 Summary of Mitigation Strategies

Strategy	Role in limiting transmission	Considerations for implementation
Wearing masks (surgical, fabric)	The virus is spread through respiratory droplets from breathing, talking, coughing and sneezing. The mask catches the droplets before they can spread.	Requiring masks for all students and staff is most effective.
Hand-washing	Droplets containing the virus can spread to hands from coughing, sneezing or from surfaces. If a person then touches their mouth, nose, or eyes they may become infected. Hand-washing removes the virus.	Soap and water is most effective. Hand-sanitizer is appropriate to use if soap and water are not available. Minimum times for hand washing -- before and after eating, after using the restroom.
Physical distancing -- Maintaining 3 to 6 feet between students and staff	When people are in close contact they can easily breathe in droplets containing the virus that other people have exhaled. Most droplets will fall to the ground within 3-6 feet of being exhaled.	How this is implemented will depend on the number of students in the school and the size of classrooms. The key is maintaining sufficient space between students and between students and the teacher. There is no evidence about the relative effectiveness of different ways of implementing physical distancing in schools.
Eliminating large gatherings	If a person is sick, large gatherings with close contact mean that many other people may be infected.	This includes eliminating assemblies, large sports events, and large numbers of students in common areas (cafeteria, hallways, entryways)
Creating cohorts (one teacher stays with the same group of students)	Smaller groups of students in a classroom allow for more distance between people. In addition, limiting contact with many other people, cuts down on possible exposures.	Members of the cohort do not mix with the rest of the school. The teacher should also have minimal contact with students and other staff outside of the cohort.
Cleaning	Droplets can land on surfaces and remain active for 1-3 days. If a person touches the surface with their hands and then touches their mouth, nose or eyes, they can contract the virus.	Regular cleaning is important to eliminate the virus on surfaces. Routine cleaning with appropriate disinfectant is sufficient. Cleaning is particularly important for high touch areas and shared materials.
Ventilation	While most droplets containing the virus fall out of the air, some can stay suspended. If enough suspended droplets accumulate they could be breathed in by occupants. When fresh air is added to a room where virus is present, the amount of virus is diluted or eliminated.	Small rooms with poor ventilation are likely to increase risk of transmission. Open windows and doors to increase circulation of outdoor air as much as possible. Moving classroom activities out-of-doors is also an option for improving ventilation.
Air filtering	Mechanical heating, cooling and ventilation control and regulate the amount and quality of air in buildings for humidity, temperature and particulates. For efficiency, some systems recirculate the indoor air as much as possible to reduce the energy costs of treating outside air. If there are droplets containing the virus in the air, recirculation could spread COVID within a building. Upgraded filters can remove droplets containing the virus from the air.	To provide maximum protection, upgrade the filters used in the HVAC system, increase the fresh air intake, and increase the level of humidity.
Temperature and symptom screening	The intent is to identify individuals who have COVID-19 and prevent them from bringing the virus into the building.	There is increasing evidence that people are contagious before they show symptoms. This means the considerable time and costs to screen all students before entering buses or schools may be of limited value for identifying COVID cases. Studies in airports show limited value. However, parents should know the symptoms for COVID-19 and screen their children and household for them each day before sending children to school.

Administrative Controls

As noted in the previous section, many of the mitigation strategies outlined by the CDC fall into the administrative control level of the hierarchy of controls. We have identified a set of these as particularly important to implement, given the way COVID-19 is transmitted: handwashing, physical distancing, cohorting, and avoiding use of shared instructional materials or equipment.

Routines for Handwashing and Hygiene

The CDC (2020) recommends that individuals wash their hands

- "Before, during, and after preparing food
- Before eating food
- Before and after caring for someone at home who is sick with vomiting or diarrhea
- Before and after treating a cut or wound
- After using the toilet
- After changing diapers or cleaning up a child who has used the toilet
- After blowing your nose, coughing, or sneezing
- After touching an animal, animal feed, or animal waste
- After handling pet food or pet treats
- After touching garbage
- After you have been in a public place and touched an item or surface that may be frequently touched by other people, such as door handles, tables, gas pumps, shopping carts, or electronic cashier registers/screens, etc.
- Before touching your eyes, nose, or mouth because that's how germs enter our bodies."

To make these recommendations feasible in a school setting, the committee observes that at a minimum schools will have to provide handwashing opportunities after using the restroom and before eating, along with making alcohol-based hand sanitizer available in classrooms and shared spaces such as a gymnasium or cafeteria. Providing frequent opportunities for handwashing may be especially difficult in school buildings with limited or poorly functioning restroom facilities. In these cases, hand sanitizer can be used, if improving or repairing restrooms is not possible.

Physical Distancing

Physical distancing (also called social distancing) is a key strategy for limiting transmission. Fundamentally it involves avoiding close, physical contact with other people. The CDC recommends that people keep at least 6 feet away from people outside of their household.

In the context of schools, physical distancing may require many changes to routines and use of space. Classrooms will need to be organized to allow students and the teacher to maintain distance from each other. It may be necessary to limit the number of students in the classroom or to move instruction to a larger physical space. Different staffing models will likely need to be considered depending on the particular strategy employed. In schools that are already overcrowded, creating space for physical distancing may be difficult.

Another important aspect of physical distancing is limiting large gatherings of students, such as in the cafeteria, in assemblies, or for indoor sports events. This also means avoiding overcrowding at school entrances and exits at the beginning and end of the school day, potentially by staggering arrival and departure times. The specific strategies will depend on the characteristics of each school building and the number of students in attendance.

Cohorting

Cohorting denotes having the same small group of students (10 or fewer) stay with the same staff as much as possible. This model has been used in some other countries that have reopened school buildings. For example, in Denmark class size was limited to 10–11 students to allow distancing between students and staff were limited to working with 1 or 2 classes (Melnick et al., 2020).

A benefit of this approach is that it limits the number of different people with whom any single individual has contact. This approach is likely easiest to implement in elementary schools, because elementary classrooms are already organized such that one teacher works consistently with the same group of students. In the upper grades, students typically move between classes, often mixing from class to class. Of interest, the use of small cohorts for middle school students may be more developmentally appropriate than the usual structure of students changing classrooms for every class because it offers an opportunity for developing a closer relationship with the teacher (Eccles et al., 1993).

In planning for different versions of cohorting, it is important to keep in mind that the main goal is to limit the exposure to others of *all* individuals, including both teachers and the students. Thus models whereby a teacher sees multiple cohorts of students in the same day, or across several days, may not meaningfully reduce risk for the teacher. To limit the amount of contact each teacher has with multiple different students, schools could consider creative uses of virtual instruction. For example, a cohort of students might be physically with a lead teacher, while teachers of specific subjects would join the class virtually for a period of time.

Avoiding Use of Shared Materials and Equipment

Because of the risk of transmission from surfaces, it is important to minimize shared objects such as manipulatives used in teaching, art supplies, or technology. If they are shared, they need to be cleaned between uses (see section on cleaning below).

Engineering Controls

Key strategies at the engineering control level are cleaning, ventilation and air quality, and temperature and symptom screening. However, it is important to stress that implementing these strategies only is unlikely to limit transmission enough to prevent students or staff from getting sick.

Surface Cleaning

Regular cleaning is important, but schools will find it nearly impossible to clean as frequently as would be needed to ensure that surfaces remain completely virus-free at all times. Emerging evidence suggests that the virus persists on most hard surfaces for 2–3 days and on soft surfaces for 1–2 days (van Doremalen et al., 2020). The CDC has guidance on cleaning and disinfecting available that schools can use to guide their procedures (CDC, 2020). At minimum, surfaces should be cleaned and disinfected nightly.

Even with regular cleaning, it is important to minimize contact with shared surfaces such as manipulatives or other hands-on equipment in the classroom. Strategies for minimizing transmission via shared surfaces include assigning equipment to individual students to prevent multiple users, and disinfecting items between users. Use of soft-touch items that are difficult to disinfect should be minimized.

Cleaning is especially important when someone in the school building becomes sick while on site and/or tests positive for COVID-19. In these cases, the protocols laid out in the CDC guidance should be followed, including closing off space(s) where the infected person was for 24 hours if possible before cleaning and disinfecting. In many cases, this may include shared restrooms.

Air Quality and Ventilation

As noted above, the primary mechanism of transmission of SARS-CoV-2 is through respiratory droplets traveling through the air. While many of these droplets are heavy and drop out of the air, some may remain airborne for a longer period of time as aerosols (very small, floating droplets).

In a small space with poor ventilation, the droplets and aerosols in the air may accumulate enough to create a risk of infection. For this reason, it is important to ensure that classrooms and other spaces in the school building are well ventilated. Ventilation systems should be operating properly and, when possible, circulation of outside air should be increased, for example by opening windows and doors. Also, use of face masks will limit the number of droplets and aerosols that are released into the air.

Maintaining sufficient ventilation may be difficult in classrooms with windows that do not open, or in schools with poorly functioning ventilation systems. As noted in Chapter 3, poor air quality and outdated HVAC systems may be particularly problematic for under-resourced schools.

A recent report from the Harvard School of Public Health (Jones et al., 2020) identifies key strategies for ensuring air quality and proper ventilation. The report emphasizes the importance of bringing in outdoor air to dilute or displace any droplets containing the virus that may be present in the air. They also recommend avoiding recirculation of indoor air, increasing filter efficiency, and supplementing with portable air cleaners. The report's authors also stress the importance of verifying the performance of ventilation and filtration through testing and working with outside experts. These additional strategies represent additional costs to schools, but they may be especially important for older school buildings with outdated HVAC systems, or for buildings with limited ventilation.

Temperature and Symptom Screening

Temperature and symptom screening is mentioned in two places in the CDC decision tree. While it is important to be sure that people who are infected do not enter the building, there is mounting evidence that people may be contagious before they show symptoms of COVID-19. This means that screening may not identify all individuals who pose a risk for bringing the virus into the school. In addition, temperature screening alone is less likely to identify individuals than temperature and symptom screening.

Applying the Strategies to Transportation

Many districts around the country use transportation systems, such as buses, to enable safe, reliable passage to school for children. As noted in

Chapter 3, about 33 percent of students in the United States ride a school bus to get to school. A major concern for school districts is that it is impossible to transport students to schools in a school bus while maintaining a 6-foot distance between children. If buses were to reduce capacity in accordance with physical distancing guidelines, they would likely be able to transport only 8–10 students per bus at a time. Given this constraint, epidemiological wisdom points to limiting the use of buses. When their use is necessary, however, strategies include avoiding seating students in the two seats closest to the driver, disinfecting shared surfaces (e.g., hand rail, buttons) after each stop if possible, disinfecting all surfaces between trips, and for HVAC systems, using the highest setting and changing filters regularly.

A small number of students, about 2 percent, across the country, take public transportation to school. This poses additional risks of exposure over which districts have little control.

The Cost of Mitigation

The cost of implementing all of the suggested strategies is very high. The Council on School Facilities estimates that the total cost for schools nationwide could be $20 billion. A recent estimate reported by EdWeek (Will, 2020) suggests that for the average district, the cost of implementing the strategies might be as much as $1,778,139 for the 2020–2021 school year (see Box 5-1 for the breakdown of estimated costs for an average district). This estimate is based on costs for a district with 3,269 students, 8 school buildings, 183 classrooms, 329 staff members, and 40 school buses operating at 25 percent capacity.

The actual costs will vary by school district depending on regional prices, economies of scale (how much volume districts can purchase), and the availability of labor and goods necessary to comply with recommended physical distancing and cleaning protocols. The model for the transportation costs assumes running buses at 25 percent typical capacity to adhere to physical distancing guidelines. The costs do not include the extra funds needed to provide staff and students with training in the new protocols.

These extra costs for reopening for in-person learning and limiting transmission of the virus among students and staff are coming at a time when state budgets are shrinking because of the economic impact of the pandemic. This means that education budgets are being cut, making it even more difficult for districts and schools to find the funding to implement all of the necessary measures. As a result, districts will have budgetary reasons for only partially implementing the CDC's recommended strategies as well as practical ones. However, as mentioned in Chapter 4, districts and schools

BOX 5-1
Estimated Costs of Implementing Recommended
Strategies for Limiting the Transmission of
COVID-19 in Schools (for an Average District)

Health & Safety Protocols: Total = $1,232,000

Increasing custodial staff for increased cleaning/disinfecting of schools and buses to prevent spread	$448,000
Placing at least one full-time or part-time nurse in every school building	$400,000
Assigning one transportation aide per bus to screen students' temperatures (public health officials have not recommended this practice)	$384,000

Transportation & Childcare: Total = $235,144

Resume before/after-school child care programs (with physical distancing and cleaning protocols)	$168,750
Fog machines and cleaner for buses	$55,860
Hand sanitizer for buses	$10,534

Personal Protective Equipment: Total = $195,045

Disposable masks for students who do not bring their own (est. 30% of students)	$148,190
Daily disposable masks for in-school staff	$44,415
Gloves for custodial staff (5 pairs per day for two custodians per school)	$1,440

Equipment for Health Monitoring & Cleaning: Total = $116, 950

Electrostatic disinfectant sprayers	$33,600
Disinfectant wipes for classrooms (four containers per day/per classroom)	$16,833
Hand sanitizer for students in classrooms	$39,517
Deep cleaning of school after a confirmed case	$26,000
No-touch thermometer (one per school)	$640
Oximeter (one per school)	$360

Additional Costs

Physical distancing signs and markers in the building	$1,500 for districts to prepare and post signage on physical distancing in their schools and buses; $100 for each school to prepare site markings on sidewalks and play areas
Add motion-sensor dispensers for soap and water in the bathrooms.	$300 per touchless faucet, $200 to outfit each toilet with touchless controls, $50 per touchless soap dispenser, and $150 per touchless paper towel dispenser; districts might also need to upgrade their plumbing to support those installations, which would cost significantly more
Staff to monitor bathrooms	
Repurposing additions to classrooms	$7,500 for educational facilities space planners to help reorganize space and furniture in a district's school buildings
Add outdoor classrooms if possible	A one-time cost of $5,000 to $10,000 per classroom, depending on whether the district purchases a tent or canopy to protect students from sun and precipitation; districts need seating for students, some sort of covering to provide shade, portable teaching supplies such as white boards, and storage for supplies
Install plastic shields in the front office	$1,000
Repair HVAC	Major repairs for HVAC systems are estimated to cost about $3 a school building square foot, and replacements are estimated to be about $10 per building square foot

HVAC = heating, ventilation, and air conditioning (systems).
NOTE: This estimate is based on costs for a district with 3,269 students, 8 school buildings, 183 classrooms, 329 staff members, and 40 school buses operating at 25 percent capacity.
SOURCE: Association of School Business Officials International; AASA, the School Superintendents Association.
CITED IN: *This information originally appeared in Education Week on June 10, 2020. Reprinted with permission from Editorial Projects in Education.*

have little guidance on how to select which strategies might be most effective for limiting the spread of COVID-19.

Mitigation Strategies in International Contexts

As K–12 schools in the United States move toward reopening for in-person learning, it may become possible to learn about the effectiveness of strategies for mitigating the transmission of COVID-19 from other countries that have reopened their school buildings. Although research on these strategies in international contexts is nascent, understanding how other school systems have managed the crisis may provide insight into what schools in the United States can do to mitigate transmission as they reopen. Table 5-2 provides a snapshot of the strategies and methods other countries have used when reopening their schools to in-person learning.

CREATING A CULTURE FOR MAINTAINING HEALTH

The suite of strategies for limiting transmission during the pandemic will create many new routines that students and staff will need to follow and behaviors they will need to adopt. These measures will be most successful if the majority of people follow them consistently. As the CDC guidelines point out, this will require that all staff and students learn about the strategies, why they are important, and how to adhere to them as well as possible. The CDC also recommends the use of signage to remind students of the strategies and to illustrate how they can move through the building in ways that maintain physical distancing.

Providing training for all staff and students is an important part of ensuring that the strategies are implemented properly. The training should be provided by local public health officials possibly in collaboration with the school nurse. Staff and families should also receive training in how to identify symptoms and on criteria for when they, or their children, should stay home because they are sick.

Even with training and signage, staff will need to help students continue to follow these strategies. The fact that staff will need to monitor and enforce the guidelines around mask wearing, physical distancing, and handwashing opens up the possibility that patterns of enforcement of the new measures will follow the same trends that are seen in school discipline more generally. Should this be the case, Black students, boys, and students with disabilities will be particularly vulnerable to potentially harsh responses if they fail to follow the strategies consistently (Anderson and Ritter, 2017; U.S. Government Accountability Office, 2018). To guard against this, positive approaches to encouraging adherence to the strategies are preferred over punitive ones.

TABLE 5-2 Summary of Health and Safety Practices in International Contexts

	China	Denmark	Norway	Singapore	Taiwan
Context	Gradual reopening since March	Opened April 15 for children up to age 12	Opened April 27 for Grades 1–4	Opened until April 8, then closed due to non-school-related outbreak	Never fully closed; local, temporary closures as needed
Health screening	Temperature and symptoms checks at least twice daily	Temperature and symptoms checks on arrival	Temperature and symptoms checks on arrival	Temperature and symptoms checks twice daily	Temperature and symptoms checks on arrival
Quarantine and school closure policy	Quarantine if sick until symptoms resolve	Stay home 48 hours if sick	Stay home if sick until symptom-free 1 day	Quarantine required and legally enforced if one has had close contact with a confirmed case; school closes for deep cleaning if case confirmed	Class is suspended 14 days if one case confirmed, school suspended 14 days if 2+ cases
Group size and staffing	Class size reduced from 50 to 30 in some areas of the country	Class sizes reduced to accommodate 2-meter (6 feet) separation in classrooms; non-teaching staff provide support	Maximum class size 15 for Grades 1–4, 20 for Grades 5–7	No maximum class size; classrooms are large enough to ensure 1–2 meter (3–6 feet) separation	No maximum class size; students in stable homerooms; subject-matter teachers move between classes
Classroom space/ physical distancing	Group desks broken up; some use dividers	Physical distancing (2 meters) within classrooms; use of outdoor space, gyms, and secondary school classrooms	Physical distancing within classrooms; use of outdoor space encouraged	Group desks broken up in Grade 3 and up; 1–2 meter (3–6 feet) distance maintained	Group desks broken up; some use dividers
Arrival procedures	Designated routes to classes; multiple entrances	No family members past entry; staggered arrival/ dismissal	No family members past entry; staggered arrival/ dismissal	No family members past entry; parents report travel; staggered arrival/ dismissal	No family members past entry
Mealtimes	Eat at desks or, if cafeteria used, seating is assigned in homeroom groups	Sit well apart while eating; no shared food	Eat at desks or, if cafeteria used, homeroom groups enter in shifts	Assigned seating in cafeteria with 1–2 meter (3–6 feet) spacing	Eat at desks; some use dividers
Recreation	Some schools have suspended physical education	Students play outside as much as possible; play limited to small groups within homeroom	Students sent outside as much as possible; play limited to small groups; outdoor space divided and use is staggered	Inter-school sports suspended; small-group play time staggered	Sports and physical education suspended
Transport	Using "customized school buses" with seats farther apart to limit proximity	School buses allowed; only one student per row	Private transportation encouraged; one student per row on buses	Still running buses and public transit	Still running buses and public transit, cleaning at least every 8 hours
Hygiene	Masks required, provided by the government; frequent handwashing	Frequent handwashing; posters and videos provided	Staff training on hygiene standards; frequent handwashing; posters and videos provided	Frequent handwashing; posters and videos provided	Masks required, provided by the government; windows and air vents left open

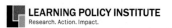 **LEARNING POLICY INSTITUTE**
Research. Action. Impact.

LearningPolicyInstitute.org
@LPI_Learning
facebook.com/LearningPolicyInstitute

SOURCE: *Reopening Schools in the Context of COVID-19: Health and Safety Guidelines from Other Countries* by Hanna Melnick and Linda Darling-Hammond, with the assistance of Melanie Leung, Cathy Yun, Abby Schachner, Sara Plasencia, and Naomi Ondrasek is licensed under a Creative Commons Attribution-Non-Commercial 4.0 International License.

Finally, ensuring that students and staff who are just beginning to experience symptoms do not come to school is one of the most important mitigation strategies that schools can adopt. To encourage this, the CDC recommends that districts and schools consider developing policies that encourage people to stay home when they are sick. For example, by eliminating perfect attendance awards for students or making sure that staff know there will not be negative repercussions if they need to stay home.

WHAT TO DO WHEN SOMEONE GETS SICK

As the committee notes, even with all of these mitigation strategies in place, it is likely that someone in the school community will contract COVID-19. The CDC provides guidelines on what to do in these circumstances. We highlight key steps here.

First, families and staff need clear guidance on symptoms of COVID-19, when to stay home, and the procedure for notifying school officials. As noted above, training for families and staff that includes these procedures will be needed. Clear guidance reminding families of the procedures should be sent to families and made available online. In addition, parents and students should have access to information, resources, and referral for COVID-19 testing sites prior to the beginning of the school year.

If someone develops symptoms at school, they need to quickly be isolated from the rest of the school population. This means that schools will need to create an isolation area and have designated staff, such as a school nurse, to monitor and care for the sick individual until they can be transported home or to a health care facility. Ideally, the isolation area will be vented to the outside to prevent droplets containing the virus to circulate in the rest of the building.

In accordance with state and local laws and regulations, school administrators will need to notify local health officials, school staff, and families immediately of any case of COVID-19 while maintaining confidentiality. They will also need to inform any individuals who have had close contact with a person diagnosed with COVID-19 to stay home and self-monitor for symptoms.

As noted earlier in the chapter, cleaning and disinfecting is especially important after someone who has tested positive for COVID-19 has been in the school. The areas used by the sick person will need to be closed off for at least 24 hours, if possible, before being cleaned and disinfected. School leaders will need to consult with public health officials about whether short-term closure of the building might be warranted (for example, if several students in a classroom, or several staff members test positive).

Students and staff who have been sick will not be able to return to the school until they have met the CDC criteria to discontinue home isolation. Caregivers and staff will need to wait for formal notification from the school nurse or a physician that it is permissible for them to return to school.

Monitoring health of students and staff and caring for individuals who become sick will place a heavy burden on school nurses and other school health staff. In schools that currently employ part-time nurses or do not have a school nurse at all, staffing will need to be supplemented. Local health departments of hospital health systems may need to partner with schools to provide nurse triage services within the school district to handle parental health calls/inquiries and to act as a referral resource for faculty and staff to maintain the optimal health of children.

CONCLUSIONS

Conclusion 5.1: The recommended list of mitigation strategies is long and complex. Many of the strategies require substantial reconfiguring of space, purchase of additional equipment, adjustments to staffing patterns, and upgrades to school buildings. The financial costs of consistently and fully implementing the strategies are high.

Conclusion 5.2: The extent to which mitigation strategies can be implemented and how will vary depending on the age of students, the physical constraints of the school building, and the resources available in the school or district. Implementing all of the recommended strategies will likely be challenging depending on the resources and the size and condition of the schools within a district. Districts that are already highly resourced and have well-maintained buildings will be more likely to be able to implement the full suite of strategies.

Conclusion 5.3: There is limited evidence about the relative effectiveness of the various mitigation strategies recommended for schools. This limited evidence base makes it difficult to provide clear guidance to schools about which strategies they may be able to relax or eliminate— given practical and cost constraints—without increasing the risk of viral transmission. Without input from outside experts, districts and schools are left on their own to make these difficult judgments.

Conclusion 5.4: Although cleaning and improving air quality and ventilation are important mitigation strategies, they are insufficient for limiting transmission of the virus enough to keep people from getting sick. Mask wearing, handwashing, and physical distancing are essential.

Conclusion 5.5: Even with all of the mitigation strategies in place and well implemented, it will be impossible to bring the risk of contracting the virus to zero. As long as the virus is present in communities, schools may be subject to transmission.

6

Recommendations and Urgent Research

Whether to reopen school buildings for the 2020–2021 school year is one of the most consequential and complex decisions many education leaders will ever have to make. While the benefits of reopening for students, families, and communities are clear, leaders must also take into account the health risks to school personnel and students' families, as well as the practicality and cost of the mitigation strategies that will be needed to operate safely. These decisions are made more difficult by the lack of definitive evidence about transmission in children or about which mitigation measures are most effective for limiting the spread of the virus in schools.

Recognizing these challenges and the difficult choices faced by education leaders, the committee offers a set of eight recommendations intended both to provide guidance as leaders make these choices and to serve as a call to action for other stakeholders to provide support for educators in this difficult time. We also offer a ninth recommendation identifying four areas of research we believe need urgent attention so that decision-makers can soon have the evidence base they need for making more informed choices.

Recommendation 1: *The Decision to Reopen*
Districts should weigh the relative health risks of reopening against the educational risks of providing no in-person instruction in Fall 2020. Given the importance of in-person interaction for learning and development, districts should prioritize reopening with an emphasis on providing full-time, in-person instruction in grades K–5 and for students with special needs who would be best served by in-person instruction.

A complex set of risks and trade-offs surrounds decisions about reopening school buildings. Reopening schools for in-person learning will necessarily bring a number of risks related to health and safety. Not reopening schools, however, also carries a number of risks that need to be considered. Distance learning, while an essential tool for ensuring continuity of instruction when school buildings are closed, cannot fully take the place of in-person interaction. Moreover, disparities in access to reliable Internet and appropriate electronic devices could compound already existing educational inequities. The risks of not having face-to-face learning are especially high for young children, who may suffer long-term consequences academically if they fall behind in the early grades.

Recommendation 2: *Precautions for Reopening*
To reopen during the pandemic, schools and districts should provide surgical masks for all teachers and staff, as well as supplies for effective hand hygiene for all people who enter school buildings.

In order to open for in-person learning, schools and districts will need to leverage the strengths and talents of teachers and school staff by attending to their health and safety concerns. As discussed in Chapter 3, a significant portion of the teacher workforce is over the age of 65, signaling that these individuals are both at increased risk related to COVID-19, *and* eligible for retirement. This reality, combined with the fact that many schools and districts may choose to limit interaction among students by assigning students to smaller cohorts or pods, poses a serious human capital challenge for education stakeholders to consider. To make returning to work a safe and desirable option, stakeholders will need to take the health and safety concerns of teachers and staff seriously.

Recommendation 3: *Partnerships Between School Districts and Public Health Officials*
Local public health officials should partner with districts to

- assess the readiness of school facilities to ensure that they meet the minimum health and safety standards necessary to support COVID-19 mitigation strategies;
- consult on proposed plans for mitigating the spread of COVID-19;
- develop a protocol for monitoring data on the virus in order to (a) track community spread and (b) make decisions about changes to the mitigation strategies in place in schools and when future full school closures might be necessary;
- participate in shared decision-making about when it is necessary to initiate closure of schools for in-person learning; and

- design and deliver COVID-19–related prevention and health promotion training to staff, community, and students.

Not only will decisions related to when and how to reopen schools for in-person learning need to reflect a school district's priorities and constraints, but also plans for reopening will need to include careful monitoring of the prevalence of COVID-19 in the community. In light of the rapidly changing circumstances surrounding what is known about COVID-19, the committee emphasizes that it is unreasonable to expect school districts to have the requisite in-house public health expertise to make ongoing decisions about reopening and operating schools.

Recommendation 4: *Access to Public Health Expertise*
States should ensure that, in portions of the state where public health offices are short staffed or lack personnel with expertise in infectious disease, districts have access to the ongoing support from public health officials that is needed to monitor and maintain the health of students and staff.

Not all school districts will be able to immediately access the appropriate public health expertise locally. In many parts of the United States, especially rural areas, public health offices may be short staffed or may lack staff with deep expertise in infectious disease. Yet public health expertise is necessary for making the myriad ongoing decisions described in this report, and it is incumbent upon states to ensure that this need is addressed.

Recommendation 5: *Decision-Making Coalitions*
State and local decision-makers and education leaders should develop a mechanism, such as a local task force, that allows for input from representatives of school staff, families, local health officials, and other community interests to inform decisions related to reopening schools. Such a cross-sector task force should

- determine educational priorities and community values related to opening schools;
- be explicit about financial, staffing, and facilities-related constraints;
- determine a plan for informing ongoing decisions about schools;
- establish a plan for communication; and
- liaise with communities to advocate for needed resources.

While public health expertise is a critical component of making smart decisions related to reopening schools, it is just one perspective necessary for outlining a plan that reflects the needs and priorities of a community. As discussed in Chapter 4, many different stakeholders are invested in K–12 education. In order to approach reopening schools in ways that reflect a community's collective values, it is critical that state and local decision makers engage a range of different constituencies in the process of delineating a plan for reopening schools and monitoring their ongoing safety.

Recommendation 6: *Equity in Reopening*
In developing plans for reopening schools and implementing mitigation strategies, districts should take into account existing disparities within and across schools. Across schools, plans need to address disparities in school facilities, staffing shortages, overcrowding, and remote learning infrastructures. Within schools, plans should address disparities in resources for students and families. These issues might include access to technology, health care services, ability to provide masks for students, and other considerations.

As this report discusses throughout, decisions around reopening schools are occurring in the context of a deeply inequitable public school system. Unless school districts directly address equity in their planning process, reopening schools during the COVID-19 pandemic will undoubtedly exacerbate existing disparities in educational access and outcomes. As part of the planning process, districts will need to understand how existing inequities (in school facilities, staffing, access to resources, etc.) are likely to interact with the lived realities of communities disproportionately affected by COVID-19, so that the plans can identify where additional resources or special considerations are necessary.

Recommendation 7: *Addressing Financial Burdens for Schools and Districts*
Schools will not be able to take on the entire financial burden of implementing the mitigation strategies. Federal and state governments should provide significant resources to districts and schools to enable them to implement the suite of measures required to maintain individual and community health and allow schools to remain open. Under-resourced districts with aging facilities in poor condition will need additional financial support to bring facilities to basic health and safety standards. In addition, state departments of education should not penalize schools by withholding statewide school funding formula monies for student absences during the COVID-19 pandemic.

The various strategies for mitigating the transmission of COVID-19 reviewed in Chapter 5 will be the primary tools used by schools to support the health of their staff and students as they reopen school buildings. This list of strategies is long and complex, and implementing them will require a substantial investment of financial and human capital resources. These considerable expenditures are coming at a time when many districts are looking at uncertain financial futures as a result of the pandemic. While the size of the funding shortfall will depend on how well resourced a school district is, many districts will be unable to afford implementing the entire suite of mitigation measures, potentially leaving students and staff in those districts at greater risk of infection. In the absence of substantial financial support from the federal government and state governments, it is likely that the communities most impacted by COVID-19 will see even worse health outcomes in the wake of reopening schools.

As noted throughout this report, districts within the same state are likely to have significantly different resources (financial, human capital, etc.) to put toward reopening schools. States will need to have a role in ensuring an equitable distribution of resources so that districts can implement the measures required for a strategic reopening in their local contexts. Further, in order to equitably support districts and schools, states should not withhold funds or otherwise penalize districts if families choose remote or distance learning options for their children in Fall 2020.

Recommendation 8: *High-Priority Mitigation Strategies*
Based on what is currently known about the spread of COVID-19, districts should prioritize mask wearing, providing healthy hand hygiene solutions, physical distancing, and limiting large gatherings. Cleaning, ventilation, and air filtration are also important, but attending to those strategies alone will not sufficiently lower the risk of transmission. Creating small cohorts of students is another promising strategy.

Although it is impossible to eliminate the risk of transmission of COVID-19 in schools completely, the mitigation strategies recommended by the Centers for Disease Control and Prevention and described in this report are showing promise for reducing transmission when implemented effectively. The lack of evidence about the relative effectiveness of different strategies, especially given the considerable costs involved in implementing them all, is a challenge for districts and schools, which are left largely on their own to prioritize which of the mitigation strategies to implement and how to make judgments about any necessary modifications due to practical constraints. The committee drew on its collective expertise and the limited available evidence to identify a few mitigation strategies that appear to show promise for districts looking to leverage limited resources.

Recommendation 9: *Urgent Research*
The research community should immediately conduct research that will provide the evidence needed to make informed decisions about school reopening and safe operation. The most urgent areas for inquiry are

- children and transmission of COVID-19,
- the role of reopening schools in contributing to the spread of COVID-19 in communities,
- the role of airborne transmission of COVID-19, and
- the effectiveness of mitigation strategies.

Children and Transmission of COVID-19

The fact that as of this writing there was no scientific consensus on the role of children in transmitting COVID-19—to one another or to adults—poses a serious challenge for decision-makers. Although it is known that children are less likely both to contract COVID-19 and to experience significant consequences if they do, it is simply impossible to ascertain how likely children are to transmit the disease to school staff or adults at home. Clarity on this point would offer much-needed guidance for decision-makers regarding the necessity of various mitigation measures, and could potentially alleviate considerable anxiety for adults in proximity to students slated to attend school in person. Therefore, research is urgently needed to help understand the role of children in transmitting COVID-19.

The Role of Reopening Schools in Contributing to the Spread of COVID-19 in Communities

In addition to uncertainty around the role of children in transmitting COVID-19, much of the anxiety around reopening schools relates to how schools as a large gathering place for individuals will factor into the spread of COVID-19 in a community. To date, research on this question has produced mixed results (Hsiang et al., 2020). Clarity in this area could provide further insight into what kinds of mitigation strategies might be of the highest priority for schools. As a result, research is urgently needed that looks specifically at how the reopening of schools matters (or does not) for the prevalence of COVID-19.

The Role of Airborne Transmission of COVID-19

In the process of writing this report, the committee repeatedly returned to conversations around the role of airborne transmission of COVID-19. As described in Chapter 3, indoor air quality in U.S. public schools is notoriously poor, which can have innumerable deleterious health impacts on students and staff. However, because there is not yet scientific consensus on the role of airborne transmission in the spread of the virus, it is also unclear how the indoor air quality of schools matters in the spread of COVID-19. Given the considerable cost associated with updating aging facilities, it is particularly important to understand the exact role of airborne transmission such that stakeholders can assess the relative value and utility of that investment.

Effectiveness of Mitigation Strategies

Although this committee was expressly tasked with assessing the effectiveness and practicality of the various mitigation strategies intended to reduce the transmission of COVID-19, we were repeatedly thwarted in that endeavor by the lack of clarifying evidence. If this committee of experts was unable to reach consensus on the best direction for schools, it is likely to be extremely challenging for education stakeholders to navigate the plethora of guidance documents to determine what is best for their schools and district. Research on the effectiveness of mitigation strategies and their specific utility in school settings is needed immediately. The committee also suggests that as schools reopen to in-person learning in Fall 2020, researchers leverage the occasion to conduct research in real time, and provide guidance as soon as it becomes available.

Epilogue

The committee completed this report against the backdrop of a nation responding to the multiple deaths of Black people from police violence. In the middle of the COVID-19 pandemic, individuals of all races took to the streets in protest, demanding accountability for a broken system. Although this committee was not tasked with commenting on issues around racial justice, it is impossible to make recommendations related to reopening schools without acknowledging the larger circumstances in which many Black and Indigenous people and communities of color develop distrust of state systems.

It is within this context that the committee grappled with what to recommend to education stakeholders, and we struggled to uncover a number of unarticulated assumptions about what is best for children. In the process, we took on a series of challenging questions: What is meant when one discusses the physical and emotional safety of K–12 students? What is the role and value of schools in communities? If the United States moves to reopen schools in Fall 2020, who will truly bear the risks of this pandemic, and what does that mean for different kinds of communities across the country?

The reality, of course, is that the answers to these questions largely depend on the values and priorities of the asker. As Dr. Megan Bang of Northwestern University said in her presentation to the committee, the conclusions one draws about the evidence before them are never neutral. The logic used in deciding when and how to reopen schools reflects values and assumptions, both of which are historically situated and subject to visible and invisible power dynamics. Moreover, those values and assumptions are legible to the communities of people who go to, work at, and send their children to schools. When policy makers leave those values and assumptions uninterrogated in the face of systemic racism, they tend to crystallize into policy that reproduces pernicious deficit ideologies about communities of color. In essence, race and class *matter* in every aspect of these decisions, regardless of whether decision makers acknowledge them.

As the nation struggles to find a road to recovery in the face of the twin challenges of the COVID-19 pandemic and the epidemic of systemic racism, there are no easy answers, no quick and affordable policy decisions that will enable children to reenter schools safely while simultaneously addressing the profound systemic inequities this moment in time has laid bare. Addressing these challenges will require the coordinated and concerted efforts of all sectors in the United States. It will require commitments to equitable school financing, to engaging communities in the complicated and emotional decision-making related to reopening schools, and to centering equity in the discussions that surround those decisions.

Amid all these discourses, though, the committee sees an opportunity to use this moment as way forward in U.S. schooling. Communities across the country have a chance to consider explicitly their expectations for what roles schools should serve and to reopen schools in accordance with those priorities. Beyond the necessary investments from federal and state governments, school districts can be positioned to engage deliberately with students, families, staff, and other community interests, taking seriously their expressed needs, hopes, anxieties, and goals. With careful consideration and commitments, this can be a moment to do more than simply reopen the doors to U.S. schools; it can also be a moment to reimagine their possibilities.

References

CHAPTER 1

National Academies of Sciences, Engineering, and Medicine. (2017). *Communities in Action: Pathways to Health Equity*. Washington, DC: The National Academies Press. https://doi.org/10.17226/24624.

CHAPTER 2

Bailey, L.C., Razzaghi, H., Burrows, E.K., Bunnell, H.K., Camacho, P.E.F., Christakis, D.A., Eckrich, D., Kitzmiller, M., Lin, S.M., Magnusen, B.C., Newland, J., Pajor, N.M., Ranade, D., Rao, S., Sofela, O., Zahner, J., Bruno, C., and Forrest, C.B. (2020). *Multi-Center Observational Study of 17,148 Pediatric Patients Tested for SARS-CoV-2 Virus across the United States: A Report from PEDSnet*.

Bi, Q., Wu, Y., Mei, S., Ye, C., Zou, X., Zhang, Z., Bi, Q., Wu, Y., Mei, S., Ye, C., Zou, X., Zhang, Z., Liu, X., Wei, L., Truelove, S.A., Zhang, T., Gao, W., Cheng, C., Tang, X., Wu, X., Wu, Y., Sun, B., Huang, S., Sun, Y., Zhang, J., Ma, T., Lessler, J., and Feng, T. (2020). Epidemiology and transmission of COVID-19 in 391 cases and 1,286 of their close contacts in Shenzhen, China: A retrospective cohort study. *The Lancet Infectious Diseases*. Available: https://www.thelancet.com/journals/laninf/article/PIIS1473-3099(20)30287-5/fulltext.

Castagnoli, R., Votto, M., Licari, Castagnoli, R., Votto, M., Licari, A., Brambilla, I., Bruno, R., Perlini, S., Rovida, F., Baldanti, F., and Marseglia, G.L. (2020). Severe acute respiratory syndrome coronavirus 2 (SARS-CoV-2) infection in children and adolescents: A systematic review. *JAMA Pediatrics*. Published online April 22, 2020. https://doi.org/10.1001/jamapediatrics.2020.1467.

Centers for Disease Control and Prevention. (2020a). *Cases, Data, and Surveillance. A Weekly Surveillance Summary of U.S. COVID-19 Activity*. (Updated July 1). Available: https://www.cdc.gov/coronavirus/2019-ncov/cases-updates/index.html.

_____. (2020b). *Community, Work & School: Considerations for Schools.* (Updated May 19). Available: https://www.cdc.gov/coronavirus/2019-ncov/community/schools-childcare/schools.html.

_____. (2020c). *Cases, Data, and Surveillance. COVIDView Weekly Summary.* (Updated July 3). Available: https://www.cdc.gov/coronavirus/2019-ncov/covid-data/covidview/index.html.

_____. (2020d). *Community, Work & School: General Business Frequently Asked Questions.* (Updated May 3). Available: https://www.cdc.gov/coronavirus/2019-ncov/community/general-business-faq.html.

_____. (2020e). *Your Health: People Who Are at Higher Risk for Severe Illness.* (Updated June 25). Available: https://www.cdc.gov/coronavirus/2019-ncov/need-extra-precautions/people-at-higher-risk.html.

DeBiasi, R.L., Song, X., Delaney, M., Bell, M., Smith, K., Pershad, J., Ansusinha, E., Hahn, A., Hamdy, R., Harik, N., Hanisch, B., Jantausch, B., Koay, A., Steinhorn, R., Newman, K., and Wessel, D. (2020). Severe COVID-19 in children and young adults in the Washington, DC, metropolitan region. *The Journal of Pediatrics.* https://doi.org/10.1016/j.jpeds.2020.05.007.

Gostic, K.M., Kucharski, A.J., and Lloyd-Smith, J.O. (2015). Effectiveness of traveller screening for emerging pathogens is shaped by epidemiology and natural history of infection. *ELife.* https://doi.org/10.7554/eLife.05564.

Inglesby, T.V. (2020). Public health measures and the reproduction number of SARS-CoV-2. *JAMA Insights.* https://doi.org/10.1001/jama.2020.7878.

Jing, Q.L., Liu, M.J., Yuan, J., Zhang, Z.B., Zhang, A.R., Dean, N.E., Jing, Q.L., Liu, M.J., Zhang, Z.B., Dean, N.E., Luo, L., Ma, M., Longin, I., Kenah, E., Lu, Y., Ma, Y., Fang, N.J., Yang, Z.C., and Yang, Y. (2020). Household secondary attack rate of COVID-19 and associated determinants. *medRxiv.* https://doi.org/10.1101/2020.04.

Kelvin, A.A., and Halperin, S. (2020). Covid-19 in children: The link in the transmission chain. *The Lancet Infectious Diseases.* https://doi.org/10.1016/S1473-3099(20)30236-X.

Li, W., Zhang, B., Lu, J., Liu, S., Chang, Z., Peng, C., Liu, X., Zhang, B., Ling, Y., Tao, K., and Chen, J. (2020). Characteristics of household transmission of COVID-19. *Clinical Infectious Diseases.* https://doi.org/10.1093/cid/ciaa450.

Lu, X., Zhang, L., Du, H., Zhang, J., Li, Y.Y., Qu, J., Zhang, W., Wang, J., Bao, S., Li, Y., Wu, C., Liu, H., et al. (2020). SARS-CoV-2 infection in children. *New England Journal of Medicine.* https://doi.org/10.1056/NEJMc2005073.

Ludvigsson, J.F. (2020). Systematic review of COVID-19 in children shows milder cases and better prognosis than adults. *Acta Paediatrica.* https://doi.org/ 10.1111/apa.15270.

NYC Department of Health and Mental Hygiene. (2020). *Percent of patients testing positive for COVID-19 by ZIP code in New York City as of April 24, 2020.* New York: Author. Available: https://www1.nyc.gov/assets/doh/downloads/pdf/imm/covid-19-data-map-04242020-1.pdf.

Prather, K.A., Wang, C.C., and Schooley, R.T. (2020). Reducing transmission of SARS-CoV-2. *Science.* https://doi.org/10.1126/science.abc6197.

Rasmussen, S.A., and Thompson, L.A. (2020). Coronavirus disease 2019 and children: What pediatric health care clinicians need to know. *JAMA Pediatrics.* https://doi.org/10.1001/jamapediatrics.2020.1224.

Resolve to Save Lives: An Initiative of Vital Strategies. (2020). *Box It In: Next Steps for Reopening Society.* New York: Vital Strategies. Available: https://resolvetosavelives.org/timeline/box-it-in.

Stokes, E.K., Zambrano, L.D., Anderson, K.N., Marder, E.P., Raz, K.M., Felix, S.E.B., Tie, Y., and Fullerton, K.E. (2020). Coronavirus disease 2019 case surveillance—United States, January 22–May 30, 2020. *Morbidity and Mortality Weekly Report.* http://doi.org/10.15585/mmwr.mm6924e2.

U.S. Department of Health and Human Services. (2020). Coronavirus disease 2019 in children—United States, February 12–April 2, 2020. *Morbidity and Mortality Weekly Report.* http://doi.org/10.15585/mmwr.mm6914e4.

U.S. Food and Drug Administration. (2020). *Coronavirus Treatment Acceleration Program (CTAP).* Washington, DC: Author. Available: https://www.fda.gov/drugs/coronavirus-covid-19-drugs/coronavirus-treatment-acceleration-program-ctap.

Verdoni, L., Mazza, A., Gervasoni, A., Martelli, L., Ruggeri, M., Ciuffreda, M., Bonanomi, E., and D'Antiga, L. (2020). An outbreak of severe Kawasaki-like disease at the Italian epicentre of the SARS-CoV-2 epidemic: An observational cohort study. *The Lancet.* https://doi.org/10.1016/S0140-6736(20)31103-X.

World Health Organization. (2019). *Non-pharmaceutical Public Health Measures for Mitigating the Risk and Impact of Epidemic and Pandemic Influenza.* Geneva, Switzerland: Author. Available: https://www.who.int/influenza/publications/public_health_measures/publication/en.

Zachariah, P., Johnson, C.L., Halabi, K.C., Ahn, D., Sen, A.I., Fischer, A., Banker, S.L., Giordano, M., Manice, C.S., Diamond, R., Sewell, T.B., Schweickert, A.J., Babineau, J.R., et al. (2020). Epidemiology, clinical features, and disease severity in patients with coronavirus disease 2019 (COVID-19) in a children's hospital in New York City, New York. *JAMA Pediatrics.* https://doi.org/10.1001/jamapediatrics.2020.2430.

Zhang, J., Litvinova, M., Liang, Y., Wang, Y., Wang, W., Zhao, S., Wu, Q., and Merler, S., Viboud, C., Vespignani, A., Ajelli, M., and Yu, H. (2020). Changes in contact patterns shape the dynamics of the COVID-19 outbreak in China. *Science.* https://doi.org/10.1126/science.abb8001.

CHAPTER 3

Alexander, D., and Lewis, L. (2014). *Condition of America's Public School Facilities: 2012–13.* NCES #2014-022. Washington, DC: National Center for Education Statistics, U.S. Department of Education.

Allen, J.G., Eitland, E., Klingensmith, L., MacNaughton, P., Cendeno Laurent, J., Spengler, J., and Bernstein, A. (2017). *Schools for Health: How School Buildings Influence Student Health, Thinking, and Performance.* Cambridge, MA: Harvard T.H. Chan School of Public Health.

American Academy of Pediatrics. (2020). *COVID-19 Planning Considerations: Guidance for School Re-entry.* Itasca, IL: Author.

American Enterprise Institute. (2020). *School District Responses to the COVID-19 Pandemic: Round 6, Ending the Year of School Closures.* Washington, DC: Author.

Bohrnstedt, G., Kitmitto, S., Ogut, B., Sherman, D., and Chan, D. (2015). *School Composition and the Black–White Achievement Gap: Methodology Companion.* NCES #2015-032. Washington, DC: National Center for Education Statistics, U.S. Department of Education.

Bureau of Labor Statistics. (2018). A look at elementary and secondary school employment on the Internet. *The Economics Daily.* Available: https://www.bls.gov/opub/ted/2018/a-look-at-elementary-and-secondary-school-employment.htm.

Cellini, S.R., Ferreira, F., and Rothstein, J. (2010). The value of school facility investments: Evidence from a dynamic regression discontinuity design. *The Quarterly Journal of Economics.* https://doi.org/10.1162/qjec.2010.125.1.215.

Clotfelter, C.T., Ladd, H.F., Vigdor, J.L., and Wheeler, J. (2007). High poverty schools and the distribution of teachers and principals. *North Carolina Law Review, 85*(5), 1345–1380.

Conlin, M. and Thompson, P.N. (2017). Impacts of new school facility construction: An analysis of a state-financed capital subsidy program in Ohio. *Economics of Education Review, 59*(C), 13–28.

EdTrust and Digital Promise. (2020). *With Schools Closed and Distance Learning the Norm, How Is Your District Meeting the Needs of Its Students? Ten Questions for Equity Advocates to Ask About Distance Learning.* Washington, DC: Author. Available: https://edtrust.org/resource/10-questions-for-equity-advocates-to-ask-about-distance-learning.

Federal Highway Administration. (2019). *Children's Travel to School: 2017 National Household Travel Survey.* FHWA NHTS Brief. Available: https://nhts.ornl.gov/assets/FHWA_NHTS_%20Brief_Traveltoschool_032519.pdf.

Filardo, M. (2016). *State of Our Schools: America's K–12 Facilities 2016.* Washington, DC: 21st Century School Fund.

Filardo, M., Vincent, J.M., and Sullivan, K. (2019). How crumbling school facilities perpetuate inequality. *Phi Delta Kappan.* https://doi.org/10.1177/0031721719846885.

Filardo, M., Vincent, J.M., Sung, P., and Stein, T. (2006). *Growth and Disparity: A Decade of U.S. Public School Construction.* Washington, DC: Building Educational Success Together.

Gross, B., and Opalka, A. (2020). *Too Many Schools Leave Learning to Chance During the Pandemic.* Bothell, WA: Center on Reinventing Public Education, University of Washington.

Hanushek, E.A., and Rivkin, S.G. (2006). *School Quality and the Black–White Achievement Gap.* NBER Working Paper #12651. Cambridge, MA: National Bureau of Economic Research. Available: http://www.nber.org/papers/w12651.pdf.

Kober, N., and Rentner, D.S. (2020). *History and Evolution of Public Education in the U.S.* Washington, DC: Center on Education Policy.

Learning Policy Institute. (2018). *Understanding Teacher Shortages: 2018 Update.* Palo Alto, CA: Author.

Martorell, P., Stange, K., and McFarlin, I. (2016). Investing in schools: Capital spending, facility conditions, and student achievement. *Journal of Public Economics, 40*(C), 13–29.

Maxwell, L.E. (2016). School building condition, social climate, student attendance and academic achievement: A mediation model. *Journal of Environmental Psychology.* https://doi.org/10.1016/j.jenvp.2016.04.009.

McFarland, J., Hussar, B., Zhang, J., Wang, X., Wang, K., Hein, S., Diliberti, M., Forrest, E., Cataldi, E., Bullock Mann, F., and Barmer, A. (2019). *The Condition of Education 2019.* NCES #2019-144. Washington, DC: National Center for Education Statistics, U.S. Department of Education.

Nagler, M., Piopiunik, M., and West, M. (2017). Weak markets, strong teachers: Recession at career start and teacher effectiveness. *Journal of Labor Economics.* https://doi.org/10.1086/705883.

National Academies of Sciences, Engineering, and Medicine. (2019a). *Monitoring Educational Equity.* Washington, DC: The National Academies Press. https://doi.org/10.17226/25389.

_____. (2019b). *Shaping Summertime Experiences: Opportunities to Promote Healthy Development and Well-Being for Children and Youth.* Washington, DC: The National Academies Press. https://doi.org/10.17226/25546.

_____. (2019c). *The Promise of Adolescence: Realizing Opportunity for All Youth.* Washington, DC: The National Academies Press. https://doi.org/10.17226/25388.

National Research Council. (1998). *Preventing Reading Difficulties in Young Children.* Washington, DC: The National Academies Press. https://doi.org/10.17226/6023.

Neilson, C.A., and Zimmerman, S.D. (2014). The effect of school construction on test scores, school enrollment, and home prices. *Journal of Public Economics.* https://doi.org/10.1016/j.jpubeco.2014.08.002.

Office of Civil Rights, U.S. Department of Education. (2014). *Dear Colleague Letter: Resource Comparability.* Washington, DC: Author. Available: https://www2.ed.gov/about/offices/list/ocr/letters/colleague-resourcecomp-201410.pdf.

Owens, A., Reardon, S.F., and Jencks, C. (2016). Income segregation between schools and school districts. *American Educational Research Journal, 53*(4), 1159–1197.

Phelps, C., and Sperry, L.L. (2020, June 11). Children and the COVID-19 pandemic. *Psychological Trauma: Theory, Research, Practice, and Policy.* Advance online publication. http://dx.doi.org/10.1037/tra0000861.

Rachfal, C.L., and Gilroy, A.A. (2019). *Broadband Internet Access and the Digital Divide: Federal Assistance Programs.* Washington, DC: Congressional Research Service.

Taie, S., and Goldring, R. (2020). *Characteristics of Public and Private Elementary and Secondary School Teachers in the United States: Results from the 2017–18 National Teacher and Principal Survey First Look.* NCES #2020-142. Washington, DC: National Center for Education Statistics, U.S. Department of Education.

Uline, C., and Tschannen-Moran, M. (2008). The walls speak: The interplay of quality facilities, school climate, and student achievement. *Journal of Educational Administration.* https://doi.org/10.1108/09578230810849817.

U.S. Government Accountability Office. (2020). *School Districts Frequently Identified Multiple Building Systems Needing Updates or Replacement.* Washington, DC: Author.

Will, M. (2020, May 9). Are teachers and principals in your state at high risk for COVID-19?: See analysis. *Education Week.* Available: https://blogs.edweek.org/edweek/District_Dossier/2020/05/how_many_teachers_and_principals_high_risk_covid_19_each_state.html.

Willgerodt, M.A., Brock, D.M., and Maughan, E.D. (2018). Public school nursing practice in the United States. *The Journal of School Nursing.* https://doi.org/10.1177/1059840517752456.

CHAPTER 4

Centers for Disease Control and Prevention. (2020a). *Interim Guidance for Administrators of U.S. K–12 Schools and Child Care Programs to Plan, Prepare, and Respond to Coronavirus Disease 2019.* Atlanta, GA: Author. Available: https://www.cdc.gov/coronavirus/2019-ncov/community/schools-childcare/guidance-for-schools.html.

_____ (2020b). *Schools and Childcare: Checklist for Parents.* Atlanta, GA: Author. Available: https://www.cdc.gov/coronavirus/2019-ncov/downloads/schools-checklist-parents.pdf.

_____ (2020c). *Interim Considerations for K–12 School Administrators for SARS-CoV-2 Testing.* Atlanta, GA: Author. Available: https://www.cdc.gov/coronavirus/2019-ncov/community/schools-childcare/k-12-testing.html.

Cheney, C. (2020, April 23). *'It's alarming!' Coronavirus Pandemic Hitting Rural Communities Hard.* Available: https://www.healthleadersmedia.com/clinical-care/its-alarming-coronavirus-pandemic-hitting-rural-communities-hard.

Eisenhauer, C.M., and Meit, M. (2016). *Rural Public Health.* National Rural Health Association Policy Brief. Available: https://www.ruralhealthweb.org/getattachment/Advocate/Policy-Documents/NRHARuralPublicHealthPolicyPaperFeb2016.pdf.aspx?lang=en-US.

National Research Council. (1996). *Understanding Risk: Informing Decisions in a Democratic Society.* Washington, DC: National Academy Press. https://doi.org/10.17226/5138.

Southern Regional Education Board. (2020). *K–12 Playbook in Progress: Considering Strategies for Reopening Schools.* Atlanta, GA: Author. Available: https://www.sreb.org/k12playbook.

Vohs, K.D., Baumeister, R.F., Schmeichel, B.J., Twenge, J.M., Nelson, N.M., and Tice, D.M. (2008). Making choices impairs subsequent self-control: A limited-resource account of decision making, self-regulation, and active initiative. *Journal of Personality and Social Psychology.* https://doi.org/10.1037/0022-3514.94.5.883.

CHAPTER 5

Anderson, K.P., and Ritter, G.W. (2017). Disparate use of exclusionary discipline: Evidence on inequities in school discipline from a U.S. state. *Education Policy Analysis Archives.* https://doi.org/10.14507/epaa.25.2787.

Centers for Disease Control and Prevention. (2020). *Reopening Guidance for Cleaning and Disinfecting Public Spaces, Workplaces, Businesses, Schools, and Homes.* Atlanta, GA: Author. Available: https://www.cdc.gov/coronavirus/2019-ncov/community/reopen-guidance.html.

Eccles, J., Midgley, C., Wigfield, A., Buchanan, C.M., Reuman, D., Flanagan, C., and MacIver, D. (1993). Development during adolescence: The impact of stage-environment fit on young adolescents' experiences in schools and in families. *American Psychologist, 48*(2), 90–101.

Jones, E., Young, A., Clevenger, K., Salimifard, P., Wu, E., Lahaie Luna, M., Lahvis, M., Lang, J., Bliss, M., Azimi, P., Cedeno-Laurent, J., Wilson, C., and Allen J. (2020). *Healthy Schools: Risk Reduction Strategies for Reopening Schools.* Cambridge, MA: Harvard T.H. Chan School of Public Health.

Melnick, H., and Darling-Hammond, L. (with Leung, M., Yun, C., Schachner, A., Plasencia, S., and Ondrasek, N.). (2020). *Reopening Schools in the Context of COVID-19: Health and Safety Guidelines from Other Countries Policy Brief.* Palo Alto, CA: Learning Policy Institute.

The National Institute for Occupational Safety and Health (2020). The Heirarchy of Controls. (Updated January 13, 2015). Available: https://www.cdc.gov/niosh/topics/hierarchy/default.html.

Perencevich, E.N., Diekema, D.J., and Edmond, M.B. (2020). Moving personal protective equipment into the community: Face shields and containment of COVID-19. *Journal of the American Medical Association.* https://doi.org/10.1001/jama.2020.7477.

U.S. Government Accountability Office. (2018). *K–12 Education: Discipline Disparities for Black Students, Boys, and Students with Disabilities.* GAO #18-258. Washington, DC: Author.

van Doremalen, N., Bushmaker, T., Morris, D.H., Holbrook, M.G., Gamble, A., Williamson, B.N., Tamin, A., Harcourt, J.L., Thornburg, N.J., Gerber, S.I., Lloyd-Smith, J.O., de Wit, E., and Munster, V.J. (2020). Aerosol and surface stability of SARS-CoV-2 as compared with SARS-CoV-1. *The New England Journal of Medicine, 382*(16), 1564–1567. 10.1056/NEJMc2004973.

Will, M. (2020). What needs to change inside school buildings? *EdWeek.* Available: https://www.edweek.org/ew/articles/2020/06/11/what-needs-to-change-inside-school-buildings.htm.

CHAPTER 6

Hsiang, S., Allen, D., Annan-Phan, S., Bell, K., Bolliger, I., Chong, T., Druckenmiller, H., Yue Huang, L., Hultgren, A., Krasovich, E., Lau, P., Lee, J., Rolf, E., Tseng, J., and Wu, T. (2020). The effect of large-scale anti-contagion policies on the COVID-19 pandemic. *Nature.* https://doi.org/10.1038/s41586-020-2404-8.

Appendix A

The Committee's Review
of Existing Evidence

As described in Chapter 1, evidence around the spread, mitigation, and treatment of COVID-19 is continuously emerging. Given this rapidly changing understanding of COVID-19, committee members relied heavily on their collective expert judgment in interpreting the available evidence. They also leveraged existing bodies of research—for example, on child development and schooling—to draw conclusions in areas where research specific to the impact of the COVID-19 pandemic is sparse or does not exist (such as research on the effects on socioemotional development of a sudden and long-term switch to solely virtual learning).

When reaching conclusions and developing recommendations, the committee drew on multiple streams of evidence: expert oral testimony was weighed alongside published literature as much as possible. However, it is important to acknowledge that, at the time of publication, many critical pieces of the COVID-19 puzzle are still missing. For example, there is still an incomplete picture of whether children—particularly those who are infected but without symptoms—can efficiently transmit the virus to others. Throughout this report, we have attempted to provide as much clarity as possible to the logic undergirding our conclusions and recommendations, as well as to identify additional research needs. The committee also solicited expert feedback on the effectiveness of strategies for mitigating COVID-19 in K–12 schools.

In order to obtain the evidence necessary to complete our review, the committee held three open sessions with experts from relevant areas of research. In the first open session, we heard testimony from Dr. Karen Bierman of the Pennsylvania State University, who discussed child development in responding to COVID-19. We also heard from Dr. Barbara Means, the Executive Director of Digital Promise, who addressed the potential and limitations of virtual learning. Dr. Michael Portman of Seattle Children's Hospital discussed the impact of multisystem inflammatory syndrome in children, and environmental science advisor Jerry Roseman discussed concerns around school facilities. We concluded the first open session meeting with a discussion with Dr. Stephen Pruitt, president of the Southern Regional Education Board, who offered perspective on how state leaders are making decisions related to school reopening.

At the second open session, the committee heard testimony on centering equity in addressing school reopening from Dr. Megan Bang of Northwestern University and the Spencer Foundation. Dr. Nancy Hill from Harvard University discussed the importance of engaging communities in school reopening decisions and plans. Dr. Lauren Ancel-Meyers of the University of Texas at Austin described her work modeling SARS-CoV-2 transmission, as well as her collaboration with the city of Austin to determine a framework for making decisions about when and how to reopen schools and businesses. Following the final committee meeting, we held one additional conversation with Dr. Linsey Marr of Virginia Tech, who consulted on indoor air quality and how schools should consider mitigating the transmission of SARS-CoV-2. The contributions of these experts were critical to helping the committee understand and respond to the breadth of challenges facing education stakeholders as they make decisions related to reopening schools.

In order to fully understand the long and complex list of strategies schools might use to assist in reducing transmission of SARS-CoV-2, the committee also sought input from epidemiologists and infectious disease prevention doctors. The committee asked a list of 30 experts to reflect on which mitigation strategies were most important for use in K–12 schools, and which were least useful. The committee incorporated this feedback into its analysis of how schools should prioritize and deploy mitigation strategies.

Appendix B

Guidance Documents Collected by the Committee

Federal Government	
Source	**Title**
Centers for Disease Control and Prevention (CDC)	*CDC Activities and Initiatives Supporting the COVID-19 Response and the President's Plan for Opening America Up Again*
CDC	*Cases Data, and Surveillance*
CDC	*Considerations for Schools*
CDC	*Considerations for K-12 Schools: Readiness and Planning Tool*
CDC	*COVIDView Weekly Summary*
CDC	*General Business Frequently Asked Questions*
CDC	*Interim Considerations for K-12 School Administrators for SARS-CoV-2 Testing*
CDC	*Interim Guidance for Administrators of US K-12 Schools and Child Care Programs to Plan, Prepare, and Respond to Coronavirus Disease 2019 (COVID-19)*
CDC	*People Who Are at Higher Risk for Severe Illness*
CDC	*Reopening Guidance for Cleaning and Disinfecting Public Spaces, Workplaces, Businesses, Schools, and Hones*
CDC	*Schools and Childcare: Checklist for Parents*
CDC	*Schools during the COVID-19 Pandemic (Decision Tree)*

State Governments

Source	Title
Alabama State Department of Education	*P-12 Supportive Guidance: Phase 3 Beginning June 1, 2020*
Alabama State Department of Education	*Checklist and Guidance for School-Sponsored Activities*
Arizona Department of Education	*Roadmap for Reopening Schools: June 2020*
California Department of Public Health	*COVID-19 Industry Guidance: Schools and School-Based Programs*
California Department of Education	*Stronger Together: A Guidebook for the Safe Reopening of California's Public Schools*
Colorado Department of Education	*Planning for the 2020-2021 School Year: A Framework and Toolkit for School and District Leaders*
Florida Association of District School Superintendents	*K12 Return to School Recommended Guidelines*
Florida Department of Education	*Reopening Florida's Schools and the CARES Act: Closing Achievement Gaps and Creating Safe Spaces for Learning*
Georgia Department of Education	*Georgia's Path to Recovery for K-12 Schools*
Hawaii State Department of Education	*Guidance for Reopening Schools*
Indiana State Department of Health; Indiana Department of Education	*Indiana's Consideration for Learning and Safe Schools In-Class: COVID-19 Health and Safety Re-entry Guidance*
Kentucky Department of Education	*COVID-19 Considerations for Reopening Schools Initial Guidance for Schools and Districts*
Maryland State Department of Education	*Maryland Together: Maryland's Recovery Plan for Education*
State of Montana Office of Public Instruction	*School Re-entry & Recovery after a Pandemic Event*
New Jersey School Boards Association	*Searching for a "New Normal" in New Jersey's Public Schools*
Pennsylvania Department of Education	*Preliminary Guidance for Phased Reopening of Pre-K to 12 Schools*
Virginia Department of Education	*Phase Guidance for Virginia Schools*
Washington Office of Superintendent of Public Instruction	*Reopening Washington Schools 2020: District Planning Guide*

Counties	
Source	**Title**
Fairfax County Public Schools (VA)	*FCPS Reopening of Schools: Draft Plans for Fall 2020*
Sacramento County Office of Education (CA)	*School Year Planning: A Guide to Address the Challenges of COVID-19*

Organizations	
Source	**Title**
American Academy of Pediatrics	*COVID-19 Planning Considerations: Return to In-Person Education in Schools*
American Academy of Pediatrics	*COVID-19 Planning Considerations: Guidance for School Re-entry*
American Enterprise Institute	*A Blueprint for Back to School*
The Aspen Institute Education and Society Program	*Recovery and Renewal: Principles for Advancing Public Education Post-Crisis*
American Federation of Teachers	*A Plan to Safely Reopen America's Schools and Communities*
The Brookings Institution	*Reopening Schools amid the COVID-19 Pandemic: Your Questions, Our Answers*
The Brookings Institution	*COVID-19 and School Closures: What Can Countries Learn from Past Emergencies?*
Collaborative For Academic, Social, And Emotional Learning (CASEL)	*An Initial Guide to Leveraging the Power of Social and Emotional Learning*
Council of Chief State School Officers	*COVID-19 Response: Phase 2 Restart & Recovery*
Harvard T.H. Chan School of Public Health	*Healthy Schools: Risk Reduction Strategies for Reopening Schools*
Johns Hopkins Bloomberg School of Public Health, Center for Health Security	*Filling in the Blanks: National Research Needs to Guide Decisions about Reopening Schools in the United States*
Johns Hopkins Bloomberg School of Public Health, Center for Health Security	*Public Health Principles for a Phased Reopening During COVID-19: Guidance for Governors*
Learning Policy Institute	*Reopening Schools in the Context of COVID-19: Health and Safety Guidelines from Other Countries*
National Association of Independent Schools (NAIS)	*Coronavirus (COVID-19) Guidance for Schools*

OECD	*A Framework to Guide an Education Response to the COVID-19 Pandemic of 2020*
Southern Regional Education Board	*Enhance or Establish a Local Task Force*
Southern Regional Education Board	*Funding*
Southern Regional Education Board	*Make Decisions for Calendars and Daily Schedules*
United Nations Children's Fund (UNICEF); World Health Organization (WHO); International Federation of Red Cross and Red Crescent Societies (IFRC)	*Key Messages and Actions for COVID-19 Prevention and Control in Schools*
United Nations Educational, Scientific and Cultural Organization (UNESCO), UNICEF, The World Bank, World Food Programme	*Framework for Reopening Schools*
WHO	*Considerations for School-Related Public Health Measures in the Context of COVID-19*

Equity Considerations

Source	Title
Alliance for Excellent Education	*Coronavirus and the Classroom: Recommendations for Prioritizing Equity in the Response to COVID-19*
Digital Promise; The Education Trust	*With Schools Closed and Distance Learning the Norm, How Is Your District Meeting the Needs of Its Students: 10 Questions for Equity Advocates to Ask*
The Education Trust	*Five Things State Leaders Should Do to Ensure Students Have Equitable Access to Learning Opportunities during COVID-19 School Closures*
Southern Education Foundation	*Distance Learning during COVID-19: 7 Equity Considerations for Schools and Districts*
Urban Institute	*Mapping Student Needs during COVID-19: An Assessment of Remote Learning Environments*

Facilities Resources

Source	Title
CDC	*Cleaning and Disinfection for Community Facilities: Interim Recommendations for U.S. Community Facilities with Suspected/Confirmed Coronavirus Disease 2019 (COVID-19)*
New York Department of Health	*Interim Cleaning and Disinfection Guidance for Primary and Secondary Schools for COVID-19*
Readiness and Emergency Management for Schools (REMS) Technical Assistance (TA) Center	*Disabilities and Functional/Access Needs Integration Resources*
REMS TA Center	*Incorporating Infectious Disease Planning Resources*
U.S. Department of Homeland Security Cybersecurity & Infrastructure Security Agency	*Guidance on the Essential Critical Infrastructure Workforce: Ensuring Community and National Resilience in COVID-19 Response*
U.S. Department of Labor Occupational Safety and Health Administration (OSHA)	*Guidance on Preparing Workplaces for COVID-19*
Washington State Department of Health	*Classroom Cleaning Tips for Teachers*

Journal Publications and News Articles

Source	Title
Analytical Chemistry	*Cognitive and Human Factors in Expert Decision Making: Six Fallacies and the Eight Sources of Bias*
Health Affairs	*Strong Social Distancing Measures in the United States Reduced the COVID-19 Growth Rate*
JAMA: The Journal of the American Medical Association	*The Urgency and Challenge of Opening K-12 Schools in the Fall of 2020*
The Lancet Child & Adolescent Health	*Screen Time in Children and Adolescents: Is There Evidence to Guide Parents and Policy?*
Nature Medicine	*Age-Dependent Effects in the Transmission and Control of COVID-19 Epidemics*
The New York Times	*Black Lives Matter May Be the Largest Movement in U.S. History*
The New York Times	*When 511 Epidemiologists Expect to Fly, Hug, and Do 18 Other Everyday Activities Again*

Appendix C

Example District Plans for Reopening Schools

As plans for reopening schools are finalized, it is clear that schools are unlikely to operate as they had prior to the COVID-19 pandemic. As of publication, the following school districts had issued plans for reopening schools in Fall 2020. These plans vary on a number of issues including, among others, the role of families in the decision-making process and the availability of different educational options for students and families.

FAIRFAX COUNTY PUBLIC SCHOOLS (VA)

Students will be returning to schools in August, and parents have already received an enrollment letter to choose how their children will go to the school for the entire year. Parents and families must submit their choices by July 10, 2020. The first option is full-time online instruction for the year with 4 days of teacher-directed instruction and 1 day of independent learning. Elementary students will receive 2.5–3.5 hours of direct instruction, while middle and high schools would attend eight periods daily. The second option is that students can attend schools in person for at least 2 days per week and engage in independent study on days they are not in schools. If families do not submit their enrollment choice by July 10th, their students will automatically be enrolled for in-person instruction (FCPS Plan for Return to School, 2020).

WASHINGTON COUNTY SCHOOLS (TN)

Schools are opening on August 3, 2020, and the county has three options to choose from when reopening. The availability of these options will depend on the rate of positive cases and what the local health department recommends at the time of reopening. The first option is a full reopening of schools with all students and staff present. This will only be approved if health officials report a flat or declining rate of cases AND recommend a full reopening. The second option is a staggered schedule where about 25 percent of students and all staff members will be present in school at one given time. Students will be present for full instruction in schools 1 day a week and will be given the necessary technology like Chromebooks to complete independent study at home. The third option is entirely virtual, where no students are physically present in schools, but professional staff are present during regular school hours. Students will have two different learning platforms available depending on their grade level for active instruction, 5 days a week. Teachers are in their classroom and available to their students electronically during the day through multiple digital platforms. All students will be assigned an email address for the school year which will be their primary form of communication. Parents and families will be able to communicate with schools through group texts, notifications from school- and teacher-approved digital applications, and the county website (WCDE School Reopening Plan, 2020).

THE SCHOOL DISTRICT OF OSCEOLA COUNTY (FL)

Schools are opening on August 10, 2020, and parents must choose between three options on how their children will attend school by July 15, 2020. The first option is a return to in-person learning. Students will commit to following safety guidelines outlined by the district, and to following the appropriate physical distancing measures. The second option is digital learning with the student's assigned school. Students will follow the traditional schedule at home with live and recorded sessions. Students may have the option to return to in-person instruction if a vaccine becomes available or conditions improve. The third option is enrolling with Osceola Virtual School, where students will engage in full-time independent learning online and also have the option to work during nontraditional school hours (Osceola *Ready. Set. Start Smart!*, 2020).

REFERENCES

Fairfax County Public Schools. (2020). *FCPS Plan for Return to School.* Available: https://www.fcps.edu/return-school/reopening-schools-plan-complete-information.

The School District of Osceola County, Florida. (2020). *Osceola Ready. Set. Start Smart!* Available: https://www.osceolaschools.net/startsmart.

Washington County Schools. (2020). *WCDE School Reopening Plan.* Available: https://www.wcde.org/cms/lib/TN02209007/Centricity/Domain/419/Reopening_Plan_7_2_2020.pdf.

Appendix D

Biographical Sketches of Committee Members and Staff

ENRIQUETA C. BOND (*Chair*) is a founding partner of QE Philanthropic Advisors, which provides consulting services for philanthropic and nonprofit organizations on program development and governance. She previously served as president of the Burroughs Wellcome Fund, a private foundation whose mission is to advance the medical sciences through the support of research and education. Prior to her role at Burroughs Wellcome, she served as a staff officer, division director, and executive officer at the Institute of Medicine (now the National Academy of Medicine). She has served on the board of the Research Triangle Park Foundation, the National Institute for Statistical Sciences, the Northeast Biodefense Center, and the New England Center of Excellence in Biodefense and Emerging Infectious Diseases. She is a member of the council of the National Institute of Child Health and Human Development, and she has served as the vice chair of the Board of Scientific Counselors for the National Center for Infectious Diseases at the Centers for Disease Control and Prevention and as the chair of the Board of Regents of the National Library of Medicine. She is a member of the National Academy of Medicine and a fellow of the American Association for the Advancement of Science. She has an A.B. from Wellesley College, an M.A. from the University of Virginia, and a Ph.D. in genetics and molecular biology from Georgetown University.

DIMITRI CHRISTAKIS is the George Adkins Professor of Pediatrics at the University of Washington School of Medicine, director of the Center for Child Health, Behavior and Development at Seattle Children's Research Institute, and an attending pediatrician at Seattle Children's Hospital. With support from the National Institutes of Health, the National Science Foundation, and numerous foundations, his laboratory focuses on the effects of environmental influences on children's health. His goal is to develop actionable strategies to optimize children's cognitive, social, and emotional development. That work has taken him from the examination room to the community and, most recently, to the cages of newborn mice. He is the author of more than 230 original research articles, a textbook of pediatrics, and *The Elephant in the Living Room: Make Television Work for Your Kids.* He is a recipient of the Academic Pediatric Association Research Award for outstanding contributions to pediatric research over his career. He has an M.D. from the University of Pennsylvania School of Medicine and an M.P.H. from the University of Washington School of Public Health.

KENNE DIBNER (*Study Director*) is a senior program officer with the Board on Science Education at the National Academies of Sciences, Engineering, and Medicine. She has served as study director for *Learning Through Citizen Science: Enhancing Opportunities by Design* and *Science Literacy: Concepts, Contexts, and Consequences,* as well as a recently completed assessment of NASA's Science Mission Directorate's education portfolio. Prior to this position, she worked as a research associate at Policy Studies Associates, Inc., where she conducted evaluations of education policies and programs for government agencies, foundations, and school districts, including an evaluation of a partnership with the U.S. Department of Education, the National Park Service, and the Bureau of Indian Education to provide citizen science programming to tribal youth. She has also served as a research consultant with the Center on Education Policy. She has a B.A in English literature from Skidmore College and a Ph.D. in education policy from Michigan State University.

LETICIA GARCILAZO GREEN is a research associate for the Board on Science Education at the National Academies of Science, Engineering, and Medicine. As a member of the board staff, she has supported studies focusing on criminal justice, science education, and climate change. Prior to joining the National Academies, she worked as a legal assistant with a law firm that specialized in security clearances and white-collar crime in Washington, D.C. She has a B.S. in psychology and a B.A. in sociology with a concentration in criminology from Louisiana State University and an M.A. in forensic psychology from The George Washington University.

MICHAEL LACH is the Assistant Superintendent for Curriculum, Instruction, and Assessment at Township High School District 113, a small district north of Chicago. Prior to this position, he served as the director of STEM education and strategic initiatives at UChicago STEM Education. He also previously served as an administrator with the Chicago Public Schools, including as chief officer of teaching and learning, overseeing curriculum and instruction in 600+ schools. During the Obama Administration, he led science and mathematics education efforts at the U.S. Department of Education. He began his teaching career teaching as a charter member of Teach for America and subsequently joined the national office of Teach for America as Director of Program Design, developing a portfolio-based alternative-certification system that was adopted by several states. In 1995, he was named one of Radio Shack's top 100 technology teachers, and he is a recipient of the Illinois Physics Teacher of the Year award. He has served as an Albert Einstein Distinguished Educator Fellow, advising Congressman Vernon Ehlers (R-MI) on science, technology, and education issues. He has a B.A. degree in physics from Carleton College, M.A. degrees from Columbia University and Northeastern Illinois University, and a Ph.D. from the University of Illinois at Chicago.

PHYLLIS D. MEADOWS is a senior fellow in the health program of The Kresge Foundation, where she advises the health team on the development of its overall strategic direction and provides leadership in the design and implementation of grantmaking initiatives and projects. She has led the foundation's Emerging Leaders and Public Health Program and advises and supports the development of cross-team programming efforts with the Detroit Environment and Human Services Programs. She is the former associate dean for practice at the University of Michigan's School of Public Health and a clinical professor in health management and policy. Her work in public health includes serving as deputy director and then director/public health officer for the city of Detroit. She has served as adjunct faculty with the School of Nursing at both Wayne State University and Oakland University. She also previously worked at the W.K. Kellogg Foundation as a program director for children and youth in education and higher education and for communities both nationally and internationally. She has a B.S.N. from Oakland University and an M.A. in community health nursing and a Ph.D. in applied sociology from Wayne State University.

KATHLEEN MOORE, the principal owner of Kathleen Moore and Associates, provides consulting services to local educational agencies throughout California. Those services cover a wide range, including educational planning, maximizing and leveraging funding, facility program management, and master plan development and implementation. Prior to starting Kathleen Moore and Associates, she was the director of the School Facilities and Transportation Services Division with the California Department of Education. In this role, she directed a staff of 40 and was responsible for the annual approval of more than 100 school sites and 400 school design plans for public school projects in California. She also provided leadership and policy development to ensure California's K–12 school facilities support student learning, achievement, and workforce development. She has a B.A. in political science from the University of California, Berkeley, and an M.P.A. from the University of San Francisco.

CAITLIN RIVERS is a senior scholar at the Johns Hopkins Center for Health Security and an assistant professor in the Department of Environmental Health and Engineering at the Johns Hopkins Bloomberg School of Public Health. Her research focuses on improving public health preparedness and response. She has participated as author or contributor to major reports that are guiding the U.S. response to COVID-19, including *National Coronavirus Response: A Roadmap to Reopening*; *A National COVID-19 Surveillance System: Achieving Containment*; *Filling in the Blanks: National Research Needs to Guide Decisions about Reopening Schools in the United States*; and *A National Plan to Enable Comprehensive COVID-19 Case Finding and Contact Tracing in the US*. She is the lead author on *Public Health Principles for a Phased Reopening During COVID-19: Guidance for Governors*, a report that is being used by the National Governors Association, the state of Maryland, and the District of Columbia to guide reopening plans. She recently testified to the House Appropriations Subcommittee on Labor, Health and Human Services, Education and Related Agencies on the COVID-19 response. She has a Ph.D. in bioinformatics and computational biology from Virginia Tech.

KEISHA SCARLETT is the chief of equity, partnerships, and engagement with Seattle Public Schools. In this cabinet-level role, she oversees all racial equity initiatives and capacity building of staff, family partnerships, community partnerships, community engagement, and strategic oversight of high-visibility, cross-organizational partnerships and philanthropic relationships. She has previously served in multiple school administration roles, ranging from STEM (science technology, engineering, and mathematics) teacher to school leader to district administrator. She is a recipient of the Middle Level Washington State Principal of the Year. She has an Ed.D. from the University of Washington.

NATHANIEL SCHWARTZ is a professor of practice at the Annenberg Institute for School Reform at Brown University. He leads Annenberg's efforts to develop local partnerships that directly improve the quality of schools and experiences of students while producing nationally relevant research. He was previously the chief research and strategy officer for the Tennessee Department of Education. In that role, he led the department's research and strategic planning teams, contributing to the launch of Tennessee

Succeeds, a strategic plan and vision aimed at increasing postsecondary and career readiness for Tennessee's 1 million students, and to the creation of the Tennessee Education Research Alliance, an innovative state-level research partnership with Vanderbilt University. He earlier worked as a high school science teacher in Illinois and Arkansas. He has a B.A. from Harvard College and an M.P.P. and a Ph.D. from the University of Michigan.

HEIDI SCHWEINGRUBER (*Board Director*) is the director of the Board on Science Education at the National Academies of Sciences, Engineering, and Medicine. She has served as study director or co-study director for a wide range of studies, including those on revising national standards for K–12 science education, learning and teaching science in grades K–8, and mathematics learning in early childhood. She also coauthored two award-winning books for practitioners that translate the findings of National Academies' reports for a broader audience, one on using research in K–8 science classrooms and one on information science education. Prior to joining the National Academies, she worked as a senior research associate at the Institute of Education Sciences in the U.S. Department of Education. She also served on the faculty of Rice University and as the director of research for the Rice University School Mathematics Project, an outreach program in K–12 mathematics education. She has a Ph.D. in psychology (developmental) and anthropology and a certificate in culture and cognition, both from the University of Michigan.

JEFFREY M. VINCENT is a director and cofounder of the Center for Cities & Schools at the University of California, Berkeley. His research and publications cover a variety of issues, including school infrastructure planning, school siting and design, sustainable communities, community development, educational economics, housing policy, state school construction policies, joint use of schools, youth engagement in redevelopment, refugee resettlement, and transportation policy. His work reflects two key ideas: that finding policy answers requires new modes of scholarship that draw on a variety of quantitative and qualitative methods and that it requires collaborative work between the too-often-siloed public, nonprofit, and private sectors. Much of his work involves "engaged scholarship," done for and in partnership with public agencies, nonprofit organizations and others with public interests in mind. He is an instructor and graduate student mentor in the university's PLUS Fellows Program. He is a recipient of the Berkeley Chancellor's Award for Public Service, Research in the Public Interest. He has a Ph.D. in city and regional planning from the University of California, Berkeley.